Recruitment and Retention in Minority Populations

Lessons Learned in Conducting Research on Health Promotion and Minority Aging

Sue E. Levkoff, ScD
Thomas R. Prohaska, PhD
Patricia Flynn Weitzman, PhD
Marcia G. Ory, PhD, MPH
Editors

Springer Publishing Company

The material in this volume was simultaneously published as a special issue of the *Journal of Mental Health and Aging* (Volume 6, Number 1, 2000).

Springer Publishing Company, Inc.
536 Broadway
New York, NY 10012-3955

00 01 02 03 04 / 5 4 3 2 1

Library of Congress Cataloging-in-Publication-Data

Recruitment and retention in minority populations : lessons learned in conducting research on health promotion and minority aging / edited by Sue E. Levkoff . . . [et al.].
p. cm.
Includes bibliographical references.
ISBN 0-8261-1375-3
1. Minority aged—Care—United States. I. Levkoff, Sue E.

362.6'089—dc21

CIP

Printed in the United States of America

Contents

Journal of Mental Health and Aging, Vol. 6, No. 1, 2000

Preface

Sue E. Levkoff, ScD
Harvard Medical School, Boston, MA

Thomas R. Prohaska, PhD
School of Public Health
University of Illinois at Chicago

Patricia Flynn Weitzman, PhD
Harvard Medical School, Boston, MA

Marcia G. Ory, PhD, MPH
National Institute on Aging, Bethesda, MD

Despite projections of significant growth in older minority populations in the next century, health and social scientists have little more than a surface-level appreciation of how cultural factors will shape mental and physical health outcomes. One of the reasons for this stems from the fact that most studies of health in old age focus on White, middle-class adults. Older minority adults have been hard to recruit and retain in such studies. The National Institutes of Health, with leadership from the Office for Research on Women's Health, has served as a catalyst for change in health research on older adults by mandating the inclusion of minorities and women in funded research. More aggressive measures for understanding the underrepresentation of minorities in research are required to meet the mandate. Until very recently, researchers have not consistently reported their recruitment experiences; and even when they have, obstacles were rarely discussed. There has also been little information on the advantages and disadvantages of research participation from the perspective of the participant and nonparticipant.

The articles in this issue are part of a new wave of studies designed to more aggressively address the issues of recruitment and retention of older minority adults. The authors in this issue describe work with diverse older populations including Latinos, African Americans, and Chinese Americans. They highlight the strengths and weaknesses of a wide array of research designs, ranging from small, in-depth qualitative studies to randomized, controlled behavioral interventions. And they not only discuss issues from the researcher's perspective, but also give voice to issues from participant and gatekeeper perspectives. The articles bring out common themes and factors associated with recruitment success and failure. Examples of these themes include: language as a barrier, the role of community and family as gatekeepers to participation, lack of trust in researchers and research, and the use of qualitative methodologies to uncover recruitment barriers.

All researchers would probably agree that language is a potential barrier to successful recruiting of older adults in non-English speaking population. The article by Hazuda and colleagues underscores the relationship between language skills, socioeconomic status, and assimilation within an ethnic group. Their research identified various levels of English proficiency among Hispanic groups within San Antonio that may be correlated with health status and participation in health promotion research.

Building acceptance and trust among community members was also a key theme in this group of articles. Prohaska and colleagues stressed the need to develop trust and approval among leaders and influential older adults within the church prior to successful recruitment of older African Americans for a church-based exercise program. Similarly, Hazuda noted that approval of family members was essential for the successful recruitment of older Hispanic women in community-based research. Acceptance by community gatekeepers was a central aspect of gaining community trust. Gatekeepers are community members, often serving in social service, health service, or religious organizations, who are respected by older adults and who can facilitate recruitment of participants. Researchers needed to identify these individuals and establish a good rapport with them, to gain community support for the research. McNeilly and her colleagues lay out ways to gain trust among gatekeepers and other community members, a critical feature of which was to continue involvement with the community beyond the scope of a particular intervention or grant. Levkoff and her colleagues also point to the centrality of reciprocity in gaining trust and commitment from gatekeepers. And Guo and colleagues highlight the ways in which culturally prescribed attitudes held by gatekeepers about the issue under study, for example, mental illness, can interfere with recruitment success.

The use of qualitative methods to better understand the barriers to recruitment and retention was stressed in most of the investigations. Especially popular were focus groups used prior to implementation of the research recruitment strategy. Focus groups held by the Drew/RAND research team (see article by Sinclair and colleagues in this volume) allowed investigators to identify potential barriers stopping older African Americans from participating in clinical trials. They identified distrust in the researchers and the university as well as a lack of knowledge of the research process. Similarly, focus groups helped Prohaska and colleagues to identify important information from the participant perspective about exercising that the researchers were able to integrate into their recruitment messages.

Finally, a theme among all investigations was the use of minority researchers representative of the target minority older populations. In many cases, this included the principal researchers while in others, this also included key research staff. For example, the investigation by Prohaska partnered (as a coprincipal investigator) with an African American faculty member from an historically Black institution who was highly identifiable in the target community, while the study by Leventhal mentored a more junior colleague who was also well known in the target community. This constituency-based approach to recruitment was supported across the other projects described in this body of articles.

Levkoff and colleagues integrate many of these overarching themes into their Matching Model of Recruitment which emphasizes making a collaborative match between the goals and perspectives of researchers and those of community members to facilitate recruitment. They also stress an issue that has been virtually absent from discussions of recruitment, that is, barriers to recruitment success can stem from researchers themselves and their home institutions. This model, as well as all the articles taken together, supports a broader understanding of the micro and macro factors contributing to successful recruitment and retention of minority older adults into research.

Thus this set of articles not only presents practical advice for other researchers, but also has an *emic* component that allows us to better understand how research looks to the people we are attempting to study. This insider's view has been missing from many of the discussions of recruitment and provides a more reliable picture of the cultural and psychosocial factors that shape minority recruitment and retention. We hope that the lessons learned from these investigations will serve as resource for future efforts to better represent minority older adults in gerontological research, and to close the information gap that currently exists for minority older adults.

Journal of Mental Health and Aging, Vol. 6, No. 1, 2000

A National Program to Enhance Research on Minority Aging and Health Promotion

Marcia G. Ory, PhD, MPH
Paula Darby Lipman, PhD
Robin Barr, DPhil
J. Taylor Harden, PhD, RNC
Sidney M. Stahl, PhD
National Institute on Aging (NIA)/National Institute of Health (NIH), Bethesda, MD

This introductory overview article addresses the importance of minority aging research for understanding and reducing health differentials found in older minority/ethnic populations, and highlights developments on the national level to draw scientific attention and resources to minority research. It sets one national effort, the Exploratory Centers for Minority Aging and Health Promotion (MAHP), a program sponsored by the National Institute on Aging and the Office of Research on Minority Health (NIH), within the larger context of federal efforts to promote minority health research over the past 15 years. This overview reviews the MAHP projects and lessons learned about outreach, recruitment, and retention that are critical for conducting research in older minority populations.

This issue examines a vital issue in research to promote health—the participation of hard-to-reach groups of older adults in research that addresses their physical and psychosocial needs. The focus is particularly on older ethnic minority Americans whose participation in research is vital if the U.S. is to make headway in reducing the disturbingly large health disparities among ethnic groups in this country.

In this introductory overview article we review the importance of minority aging research for understanding and reducing health differentials found in older minority/ethnic populations and highlight developments on the national level to draw scientific attention and resources to minority research. One national effort is the Exploratory Centers for Minority Aging and Health Promotion, a program sponsored by the National Institute on Aging and the Office of Research on Minority Health (NIH). While there is much to be learned about better methods to gain access to minority populations, the experience of these researchers, elaborated on in this issue, can begin to suggest some much needed solutions to these complex problems.

MINORITY AGING RESEARCH ON HEALTH: DESCRIPTIONS OF THE GROWING MINORITY POPULATION AND HEALTH DIFFERENTIALS

Population trends project that, in the near future, the size of the underrepresented minority racial and ethnic older populations will increase more rapidly than the European White population. These minority communities can no longer be underrepresented and understudied in health behavior and health promotion research. These underrepresented groups differ from the European White population on many psychosocial, cultural, and economic variables, all of which play important roles in health and functioning in later life.

For some time, a mortality crossover has been observed when comparing African American and White mortality patterns by age at death (Jackson, 1980; Otten, Teutsch, Williamson, & Marks, 1990). At younger ages the death rate of African Americans exceeds that of Whites, often by substantial amounts. However, at the oldest ages, the death rate of Whites exceeds that of African Americans. Recent research has gathered evidence both for the view that the crossover effect is an artifact of inflated report of age by some respondents (Ilo & Preston, 1997) and for the fact that the crossover is a real change in death rates (Manton & Stallard, 1997).

At first sight such a crossover, if real, might imply that a focus on minority aging is misplaced. Surely research should be concentrated where the differentials are greatest—at younger ages. However, a comparison of mortality tables (Cohen & Van Nostrand, 1995) from 1960 to 1991 reveals a different and more disturbing picture. In 1960 the death rates for African Americans exceeded those of Whites up to age 74. Beyond age 74, the death rate for Whites exceeded that of African Americans. At ages 85 and over the difference in death rate favoring African Americans was substantial. In 1960, a little over 20,000 Whites aged 85 and over died for every 100,000 Whites in the United States. In comparison, fewer than 14,000 African Americans per 100,000 over age 85 died. In 1960, at least statistically, the mortality crossover was noticeable.

More recently these mortality differences have shifted to later ages and have grown smaller (also see Manton & Stallard, 1997). By 1991, the death rate for all African Americans up to age 85 exceeded that of Whites. Among those aged 85 and over the death rate for African Americans was only marginally lower per 100,000 (14,272) than that for Whites (15,239). Therefore, in recent years, the crossover has all but disappeared.

Most disturbingly, however, the death rate for African American males aged 75 and over has increased between 1960 and 1991. The death rate for African American females aged over 85 increased marginally during the same interval. In contrast, the death rate for White males and females at the same ages has declined substantially.

Mortality differences in favor of Whites now exist at almost all ages. The major advances in prevention and treatment of late-life disease that have wrought substantial change in mortality for older Whites have barely changed overall mortality rates in older African American men. Though some evidence points to a mortality advantage for Hispanics over Whites in the later years of life (Elo & Preston, 1997), little data exist to track how that advantage has changed over time. As the Hispanic population has both grown substantially and become very much more diverse in the last 40 years, comparison of records from 1960 to the present time would be problematic. Data for change across time are similarly scarce or problematic for Asian Americans/Pacific Islanders and for American Indian and Alaska Native populations. Among other goals, the research described in this book represents an important effort to address the shortfalls in information about overall older minority groups.

CLOSING THE GAP IN HEALTH DISPARITIES: NATIONAL INITIATIVES TO ENHANCE MINORITY RESEARCH

The federal government's efforts to address disparities in health have been broad and included a number of initiatives. The landmark federal effort in minority health is linked to the 1985 Report of the Secretary's Task Force on Black and Minority Health and continues, today, with momentum from President Clinton's Racial and Ethnic Health Disparities Initiative (1998). During this period of time, the National Institute on Aging has promulgated race-based initiatives addressing disparities in health, gaps in scientific knowledge about "normal aging" in minority populations, and manpower shortages related to the underrepresentation of minorities in biomedical science in general, and research on aging in particular. Table 1 highlights some recent (post-1985) federal efforts, particularly those of the NIA, to address underrepresentation of ethnic and racial minorities in aging research and their unique health problems.

Recruiting and retaining minorities and women in biomedical research is a high priority for NIA/NIH. Training and preparing health professionals, both researchers and clinicians, is an essential component in the overall effort to reduce minority health disparities. The enormity of the problem led Congress to compel NIH to develop a tracking system for the inclusion of minorities and women in clinical research. Failure on the part of an investigator to include adequate plans for this inclusion is tantamount to losing a grant. The NIA has successfully implemented several manpower initiatives, including Supplements for Underrepresented Minorities in Biomedical Research and NIA Minority Dissertation Support. Furthermore, NIA is invested in ensuring that NIA-funded investigators are addressing issues relevant to the aging of minorities. However, regardless of the intentions of the research community, identifying and overcoming barriers to recruiting and retaining minorities is essential to the success of minority aging research.

In 1994 NIH revised the gender and minority inclusion policy to meet the requirements of the NIH Revitalization Act of 1993, Public Law 103-43. This law addresses issues of the recruitment of minorities and their subpopulations, and women, in all clinical research studies, especially clinical trials. The goal of the legislation is to increase opportunities for obtaining important information to enhance health and treat diseases for all Americans and to detect and account for gender and ethnic differences should they exist (NIH Outreach Notebook on the Inclusion of Women and Minorities, 1994). Commentaries on activities undertaken by the Office of Research on Minority Health (see article by John Ruffin in this issue), the Office of Research on Women's Health (see article by Vivian Pinn in this issue) and the Office of Behavioral and Social Research (see article by Norman Anderson in this issue) highlight the salience of minority health issues at the highest levels at NIH.

EXPLORATORY CENTERS FOR MINORITY AGING AND HEALTH PROMOTION

The Exploratory Centers for Minority Aging and Health Promotion (MAHP), funded from 1993 through 1997, were designed to conduct research and related activities aimed at improving the health status of older ethnic minority populations. The purpose of the Exploratory Centers was to create an interdisciplinary coordinated program to stimulate research related to diseases, conditions, and other factors that lead to ill health and disability

TABLE 1. Federal Racial and Ethnic Minority Initiatives: Correlation of Executive and Department Level Initiatives With NIH/National Institute on Aging Initiatives by Year

Year	Federal Racial and Ethnic Minority Initiatives
1985	DHHS Secretary's Task Force on Black and Minority Health
	DHHS Office of Minority Health Established (OMH)
1986	DHHS The 1990 Health Objectives for the Nation: A Mid-Course Review
	NIA Established Populations for Epidemiological Studies of the Elderly (EPESE)—North Carolina Initiative (RFC)
1988	NIA Symposium on Nutrition in Aging Blacks: Bio-Social Issues
1989	Bureau of the Census, The Black Population in the United States
	NIA Health and Retirement Survey (HRS) Initiative (RFA)
1990	Congressional Authorization of the DHHS/OMH
	Congress established The Task Force on Aging Research (TFAR) Public Law 101-557
	DHHS Submission of Healthy People 2000
	NIH established the Office of Research on Minority Health (ORMH)
	NIA The Health and Retirement Study (HRS)
1991	NIA Women's Health and Aging Study (WHAS)
	NIA Support of the Gerontological Society of America Publication, "Minority Elders: Longevity, Economics, and Health."
1992	DHHS Healthy People 2000 Progress Review
	NIH ORMH—Minority Health Initiative
	NIA/National Institute of Nursing Research (NINR)—Long-Term Care and Minority Aging Initiative (RFA)
	NIA Hispanic Health and Aging Initiative (RFA)
1993	DHHS Surgeon General's National Hispanic/Latino Health Initiative "TODOS"
	NIH Revitalization Act "Inclusion of Women and Minorities in Clinical Research"
	NIA Exploratory Centers for Minority Aging and Health Promotion Initiative (RFA)
1994	DHHS Healthy People 2000 Progress Review
	NIH ORMH National Conference on Minority Health Research and Research Training
	NIA/NINR/NIH Office of Research on Women's Health - Menopause and Health in Aging Women Initiative (RFA) also known as Study of Women's Health Across the Nation (SWAN)
	NIA Honolulu-Asia Aging Study (HAAS) Initiative added to the Honolulu Heart Program (RFC)
1995	White House Conference on Aging
1996	DHHS Healthy People 2000 Progress Review
	NIA Aging, Race, and Ethnicity in Prostate Cancer Initiative (PA)
1997	NIA/NINR/ORMH—Resource Centers on Minority Aging Research (RCMAR) Initiative (RFA)
1998	President's Racial and Ethnic Health Disparities Initiative
	NIA Networks to Enhance Minority Recruitment to Aging Research Initiative (RFA)
1999	NIH Director's Area of Emphasis on Eliminating Health Disparities

in older minority populations, to support research on health behaviors and their relationship to health status, and to develop and test interventions to improve health and functioning and programs of health education and outreach.

The Centers provided an environment in which experienced and junior investigators, and nonminority and minority investigators, interacted and directed research efforts focused on health and aging of ethnic minority populations. Ethnic minority populations studied within the Center Projects include Asian Americans/Pacific Islanders, African Americans, and Hispanics. Each Exploratory Center included pilot research projects, small-scale intervention studies, and an administrative core.

Table 2 shows research projects funded through this initiative. Of the six funded Centers, three focused on health and aging exclusively among older African Americans (Principal Investigators [PI] in Table 2: Allen, Leventhal, & Williams), and a fourth on Mexican American elderly (PI: Hazuda). The remaining two Centers (PIs: Levkoff & Prohaska) had a multi-ethnic study population. Several focused broadly on health and aging processes among older Americans (PIs: Allen, Hazuda, & Prohaska), while others had a more specific topical area (the Harvard Center on Culture and Aging, which studied issues of health and functioning for dementia-affected families; the Center for the Promotion of Health of Elderly African Americans, which focused on self-care beliefs and behaviors, and the Duke Exploratory Center for Research on Health Promotion in Older Minority Populations, which focused on the role of psychosocial and behavioral factors in hypertension). The core set of chapters in this issue represents the accomplishments of this initiative in terms of recruitment and retention issues.

RESOURCE CENTERS FOR MINORITY AGING RESEARCH

The challenges raised by the six Exploratory Centers for Minority Aging and Health Promotion led NIA to create a new program to fill knowledge gaps discovered by the MAHPs. In October 1998 NIA, with cofunding from the National Institute of Nursing Research (NINR) and the Office of Research on Minority Health (ORMH), launched the Resource Centers for Minority Aging Research, or RCMARs. The RCMARs, like their predecessor MAHPs, are committed to reducing minority and nonminority health differentials and their social sequelae for older persons by focusing on health promotion and disease and disability prevention. The RCMARs have a longer temporal perspective by fostering research and strategies to build a minority aging research infrastructure. A major objective is the development and deployment of science-based strategies for recruiting and retaining older minority group members in epidemiological, social, behavioral, and/or clinical research. Through unique partnerships with local communities, the Community Liaison Core tests and disseminates models for accessing older populations for social, behavioral, and clinical research.

The six geographically, racially, and ethnically diverse RCMARs are located at Columbia University, with a research and community focus upon Hispanic American elders; the University of North Carolina focuses upon rural African American elders; the University of Michigan and Wayne State University emphasize urban African American elders; the Henry Ford Health System focuses upon urban African Americans participating in a large, vertically structured managed care organization; the University of Colorado emphasizes mentoring and research for American Indian elders; and the University of California-San Francisco focuses upon Hispanic Americans, African Americans, and Asian Americans. A Coordinating Center, located at the Medical University of South Carolina, is responsible for multisite coordination and maintenance of a web page (http://rcmar.musc.edu).

TABLE 2. Description of Research Projects: Exploratory Center for Minority

Site/P.I.	Center Theme	Goals and Structure
The Drew/RAND Center on Health and Aging (DRC) W. R. Allen	Health and aging in the mostly African American older residents of South Central Los Angeles and surrounding neighborhoods	• Development and assessment of measurement tools • Role of the family • Models of health promotion • New interventions
Hispanic Healthy Aging Center H. P. Hazuda	Promotion of independent functioning in Mexican-American elderly in San Antonio, Texas	• Evolution of functioning/ stages of disability • Medical comorbidity and determinants of functioning • Targets for health promotion efforts
Center for the Promotion of Health of Elderly African Americans H. Leventhal	Common-sense models of disease and self-care practices among elderly African Americans in urban settings in New Jersey	• Social and psychological mechanisms underlying self-care • Commonsense representations of specific diseases • Relationship of beliefs and behaviors
Harvard Center on Culture and Aging S. E. Levkoff	Promotion of health of ethnic minority elders (African Americans, Chinese Americans, Latinos, and Whites) with dementia and their family caregivers in the Boston area	• Provide more effective and culturally informed care for dementia-affected families • How family characteristics and culturally based illness meanings and behaviors interact with health care
UIC Center for Health Interventions with Minority Elderly (CHIME) T. Prohaska	Amelioration of health risks for older African Americans and Latinos; clinic- and community-based health promotion interventions in Chicago, including public housing and community health centers	• Health promotion through modification of practices and behaviors such as exercise and diet • Comprised of community and academic advisory groups, support groups and research faculty
The Duke Exploratory Center for Research on Health Promotion in Older Minority Populations R. B. Williams	Identification of the role of psychosocial and behavioral factors in hypertension among older African Americans in North Carolina; interventions to lessen illness burden; includes both laboratory and community research	• How psychosocial and biobehavioral factors contribute to increased illness burden • Interventions to reduce blood pressure and improve knowledge of good health habits

Aging and Health Promotion (MAHP)

Research Projects	Recruitment and Other Core Activities
• Stroke Risk Assessment • Oral Health • Memory Disorders • Community-Based Health Screening and Assessment	• Centralized recruitment activities and participant registry • Centralized data entry and data base management • Accessible and validated survey instruments
• Determinants of Exercise in the Elderly • Adaptation to Subclinical Disability in Hispanic Elders • Depression in Mexican American Elders • Recovery After Major Surgery in Mexican American Elders	• Team approach to defining goals and sharing resources • Data management and analysis resources • Multidisciplinary perspective • Internal and external evaluations • Liaisons with health and community outreach projects
• Health Status Project: Medical History and other Indicators of Psychological Well-being and Physical Health • Ethnographic Study of Thoughts and Actions Regarding Health Practices, Vulnerability to Illness, and Health Care Experiences • Hypertension Project: A Descriptive Study of Common-Sense Views of Causes and Treatment of High Blood Pressure • Effects of Nutritional Supplement vs. Placebo on Blood and Immune Assays	• Methodological and procedural assistance • Data management and analytic assistance • Activities to attract and sustain involvement of minority students in research on aging and health
• Symptom Recognition and Help-Seeking Behaviors of Caregivers for Community-Dwelling and Institutionalized Elders with Dementia • Prospective, Longitudinal Study of Community-Dwelling Ethnic Minority Elders and Families • Health Provider Responses • Diagnosis of Dementia in Ethnic Minority Elderly: Case Studies from Medical Outpatient Settings • Developing a Culturally Informed Support Group Model for Chinese Families	• Community Advisory Committee activities • Diversity training for multicultural research team • Assistance in qualitative and quantitative research methods • Monthly research seminars • Centralized recruitment outreach and registry with common measures and controls
• Exercise Promotion of Minority Elderly in Senior Centers • Improving Exercise and Dietary Behaviors in Black Elders in Public Housing • Effects of Menopause/Health Promotion in Older Minority Women • Health Behaviors of Multiethnic Hispanic Elderly	• Provide resources for conducting research on health promotion in minority older adults • New, high-quality health promotion research • Dissemination of successful health promotion programs to community settings
• Epidemiological Relationships among Race, Hypertension, and Psychological Factors • Laboratory Study of the Association of Stress and Sympathetic Nervous System Activity, High Blood Pressure, and Sodium Retention • Exercise Training as an Intervention to Reduce Blood Pressure among Hypertensive Older African-Americans • Community Outreach and Health Education: Effectiveness of a Church-Based Educational Program in Increasing Knowledge of Good Health Habits	• Recruitment of study subjects • Convening regular meetings • Supervision of minority investigators • Dissemination of research findings • Assistance with special pilot projects

VOLUME OVERVIEW

Successful recruitment often begins with culturally and racially sensitive outreach into the communities in which minority individuals reside. The MAHP investigators faced a double recruitment challenge: the recruitment of older persons, and the recruitment of persons of color. Although personal experience is amassing, the identification of barriers to recruitment and successful strategies to recruit and retain older minorities is generally unavailable or lacking in the literature. More reports of culturally and racially sensitive approaches to outreach and recruitment of potential research participants are needed to enhance the quality of minority aging and health research.

The experiences of the MAHP investigators demonstrate the range of issues and possible solutions. Sue Levkoff, Becca Levy, and Patricia Weitzman present strategies for enhancing recruitment based on the perspective of researchers at the Harvard University Center on Culture and Aging. This article provides a general model of recruitment and retention that identifies enabling factors and barriers to recruiting ethnic minority caregivers of dementia-affected elderly. The model incorporates two perspectives (the perspective of researchers, and the perspective of ethnic minority groups) and three levels (the macro/ institutional level, the mediator/gatekeeper level, and the micro/individual level). The role of culture permeates all levels and all perspectives of the model. This article concludes with implications for designing successful recruitment and retention strategies for studies involving elderly ethnic minority populations.

Stacy Sinclair, Phyllis Hayes-Reams, Hector Myers, Walter Allen, Jennifer Hawes-Dawson and Raynard Kington describe experiences in the recruitment of older African Americans for health studies at the Drew/RAND Center on Health and Aging. The goal of this study was to explore important issues affecting the recruitment of older African Americans to a series of clinical studies. Qualitative techniques were used to identify potential barriers to recruitment and strategies for overcoming barriers. Three structured focus groups were conducted with seniors from two senior citizen centers in South Central Los Angeles. Most participants were unclear about what constitutes research and expressed discomfort with participation because of uncertainty about what would be required. Many also expressed general distrust of researchers, especially those perceived as having no long-term ties to the community. Recommendations that resulted from these data included the importance of similarity between staff and participants' backgrounds, training of staff regarding participants' other health care involvement, and distribution of information on how research will ultimately influence the lives of older African Americans.

Thomas Prohaska, Jacqueline Walcott-McQuigg, Karen Peters, and Min Li discuss stages of readiness to participate in a health promotion program for older African Americans. Based at the University of Illinois at Chicago Center for Health Interventions for Minority Elderly (CHIME), this study examined perceptions and beliefs about exercise and psychosocial factors associated with participation and nonparticipation of exercise health promotion programs for older African Americans in church settings. Recruited and nonrecruited participants are compared on measures of health status, attitudes and beliefs about exercise, and other demographic variables. The findings are discussed in terms of factors associated with transitions in stages of readiness to participate in exercise health promotion programs.

Another article explores the psychosocial factors related to retention of older African Americans in survey versus clinical trial research. Authors Shawna Hudson, Howard Leventhal, Richard Contrada, Elaine Leventhal, and Susan Brownlee of the Rutgers Center for the Promotion of Health in Elderly African Americans, describe efforts to recruit and retain the participation of African American elders into two different types of longitudinal research studies: surveys and clinical trials. Personal contacts by project staff as well as outreach by participants of the initial survey study were found to be the most effective sources of recruitment. For a clinical trial of hypertension, successful recruitment was due to aggressive interviewers and monetary compensation. This article discusses psychosocial predictors for those subjects willing to continue with the study.

Health promotion research with Mexican American elders is examined in an article by Helen Hazuda, Meghan Gerety, John Williams, Valerie Lawrence, Walter Calmbach, and Cynthia Mulrow of The Hispanic Healthy Aging Center. Using the matching model of recruitment developed by Levkoff and colleagues as a theoretical framework (see article in this issue), investigators examine factors affecting the recruitment of Mexican American elders in San Antonio, Texas, across their four studies. Micro-level factors among individual subjects, such as socioeconomic status, assimilation, and language skills, also vary by study design, sampling frame, and setting; however, characteristics of successful recruiters, such as cultural sensitivity, language skills, and knowledge of community, remained constant. The relevance of these findings for planning health promotion research with Mexican American elders is discussed and evaluated.

Laboratory research is the focus of the article by Maya McNeilly, Jaye Efland, Jannie Baughman, Paul Toth, Terry Saulter, Lekeisha Sumner, Andrew Sherwood, Patricia Flynn Weitzman, Sue Levkoff, Redford Williams, and Norman Anderson of the Duke Exploratory Center for Research on Health Promotion in Older Minority Populations. Specific challenges exist in recruiting minority populations for psychophysiologic studies. This article reports on factors affecting recruitment to a study investigating relationships between psychosocial factors (stress, racism, hostility, social support, and religious participation) and increases in hypertension risk factors. Both qualitative and quantitative methods were used, and participants were studied in a psychophysiologic laboratory and fed a controlled diet on a hospital clinical research unit. The primary purpose of this article is to identify factors facilitating successful recruitment of older African Americans into a research effort that required considerable time and patience from the participants.

The lack of acceptance of the label of dementia among Chinese American families is an example of a sociocultural barrier to recruitment and retention of minority elders. Through analysis of qualitative interview data, Zibin Guo, Becca Levy, Ladson Hinton, Sue Levkoff, and Patricia Flynn Weitzmann, have identified and explored the process of dementia label avoidance common among Chinese American families. Their chapter discusses how culturally shaped perceptions and concerns about mental and physical illness, the intrusiveness of research, and the natural course of the aging process often affect the participation of Chinese American families. They share the lessons they have learned to guide future research on these sensitive sociocultural issues.

SUMMARY: WHERE DO WE GO FROM HERE?

Although progress reported in this volume clearly demonstrates that minority-aging research is no longer a neglected area of study, there are still many unanswered questions and issues to address. In particular, the outreach, recruitment, and retention dilemmas raised here are themselves worthy of systematic evaluation to discover which methods work best for which groups of older minorities. Evaluative studies can be conducted to compare the effectiveness of different approaches, to determine the factors and conditions associated with highest levels of retention, and to assess methods which are most sensitive to the needs of ethnic elderly minorities. Finally, systematic focus on retention issues needs to jointly consider the complex influences of aging within an increasingly multiethnic and multiracial society, and the factors that are related to the different kinds of research being conducted (e.g., epidemiological vs. social vs. clinical). Issues such as this one, which present both the successes and the limitations of recruiting and retaining participants for minority-aging research, provide a step in the right direction.

REFERENCES

Cohen, R. A., & van Nostrand, J. F. (1995). Trends in the health of older Americans: United States, 1994. *National Center for Health Statistics. Vital Health Statistics 3*(30).

Elo, I. T., & Preston, S. H. (1997). Racial and ethnic differences in mortality at older ages. In L. G. Martin & B. J. Soldo (Eds.), *Racial and ethnic differences in the health of older Americans.* Washington, DC: National Academy Press.

Jackson, J. J. (1980). *Minorities and aging.* Belmont, CA: Wadsworth.

Manton, K. G., & Stallard, E. (1997). Health and disability differences among racial and ethnic groups. In L. G. Martin & B. J. Soldo (Eds.), *Racial and ethnic differences in the health of older Americans.* Washington, DC: National Academy Press.

Otten, M. W., Teutsch, S. M., Williamson, D. F., & Marks, J. S. (1990). The effects of known risk factors in the excess mortality of Blacks in the United States. *Journal of the American Medical Association, 263,* 845-850.

Office of the Press Secretary. (1998). *President Clinton Announces New Racial and Ethnic Health Disparities Initiative.* Washington, DC: White House Press Release.

Offprints. Requests for offprints should be directed to Marcia G. Ory, PhD, MPH, Chief, Social Science Research on Aging: BSR/NIA/NIH, Gateway Building Suite 533, 7201 Wisconsin Avenue MSC 9205, Bethesda, MD 20892-9205.

Journal of Mental Health and Aging, Vol. 6, No. 1, 2000

Promoting Minority Health Research at the National Institutes of Health

John Ruffin, PhD
Office of Research on Minority Health
National Institutes of Health
Office of the Director, Bethesda, MD

Amidst great gains in the health of the nation and current presidential initiatives is the reality of persistent, and sometimes substantial, differentials in morbidity and mortality among minority populations as compared with the White population. Compelling evidence that race and ethnicity correlate with dire health disparities among U.S. populations demands national attention. Minorities at all stages of life suffer poorer health and higher rates of premature death than the White population. With some conditions, such as asthma and HIV/AIDS, a good deal is known about why minority populations are the hardest hit, but less is known about how to reduce the disproportionate burden of these illnesses. With other conditions, such as cardiovascular disease, diabetes, dementia, lupus, and certain cancers, it is still unclear why minorities are disproportionately affected. Further, it is known that minorities participate far less in research protocols than do Whites, but little is known about how best to enhance the representation of minorities in behavioral and biomedical research. Supporting research that attempts to fill these gaps in basic health knowledge is paramount in the quest to uncover new scientific knowledge that will lead to better health for all Americans.

This issue is anticipated to become part of the national response to redress disparities in health among minority populations. Eliminating the disproportionate burden of ill health and disability among minority Americans will benefit the nation economically and socially. The Office of Research on Minority Health (ORMH), and NIH, in partnership with the National Institute on Aging, funded, in 1993, six Exploratory Centers for Minority Aging and Health Promotion to conduct research and related activities aimed at improving the health status of older ethnic minority populations. The Centers' purpose was consonant with the ORMH's twofold mission to:

- Support and promote biomedical research aimed at improving the health status of minority Americans across the life-span, and
- Support and promote programs aimed at expanding the participation of underrepresented minorities in all aspects of biomedical and behavioral research.

The ORMH continues to work in partnership with the scientists and program administrators in the NIH institutes, centers, and other federal agencies in support of its Minority Health Initiative (MHI). The MHI was launched in 1992 and is the rubric under which a series of multiyear biomedical and behavioral research studies and a set of training programs is being funded. The MHI agenda was formulated based on the recommendations of a fact-finding team that comprised 53 distinguished scientists and citizens who assimilated information and ideas from nearly 1,000 representatives of the biomedical community across the nation.

The goals of the MHI include increasing intramural and extramural initiatives aimed at improving minority health across the life span, developing protocols for intervention in health behaviors affecting the longevity and quality of life of minorities, and implementing programs that prepare more minorities for careers in science. To continue the momentum of the MHI and to further the mission of the NIH-ORMH, six priority objectives must be met:

- Promote the inclusion of minorities in research study populations.
- Enhance the capacity of the minority community to participate in addressing its health concerns.
- Increase collaborative research and research training programs between minority and majority institutions.
- Improve the competitiveness and number of well-trained minority scientists applying for NIH research funding.
- Develop an ongoing assessment tool for minority programs at NIH and a coordinated information system to link these programs.
- Increase utilization of NIH minority research supplements.

In summary, the ORMH is pleased to have partnerships that last beyond the life of a single grant award with (1) The Drew/Rand Center on Health and Aging; (2) the Hispanic Healthy Aging Center; (3) the Center for the Promotion of Health of Elderly African Americans; (4) the Harvard Center on Culture and Aging; (5) the University of Chicago at Illinois Center for Health Interventions with Minority Elderly; and (6) The Duke Exploratory Center for Research on Health Promotion in Older Minority Populations. The contributions of these centers in systematically examining issues related to the recruitment of older adults for participation in research studies needed to develop and evaluate effective interventions to meet their physical and psychosocial needs are filling a major void in knowledge. This research adds to an impressive knowledge base, helps us prepare for the tidal wave of aging baby boomers, and heralds advances in memory disorders, understanding disability decline, help-seeking behaviors of caregivers, modifiable behaviors impacting exercise and diet, and interventions to reduce high blood pressure.

Offprints. Requests for offprints should be directed to John Ruffin, PhD, Director, Office of Research on Minority Health, Building 1, Room 255, National Institutes of Health, Bethesda, MD 20892-0162.

Journal of Mental Health and Aging, Vol. 6, No. 1, 2000

Recruiting Older Women and Minority Members Into Clinical Trials: An Important Goal for Researchers

Vivian W. Pinn, MD
Office of Research on Women's Health
National Institutes of Health, Bethesda, MD

In recent years, efforts to improve the health of women have gained widespread public attention and assumed an unprecedented importance in both the biomedical and health care communities. With the new awareness of women's health issues, increased attention is also being given to improving the health of older Americans, of whom women constitute a majority. Indeed, as Americans live longer, research into the causes of aging and morbidity associated with aging has become a high priority for biomedical investigators.

In addition to the knowledge gaps concerning the health of women and the causes and progression of aging and its health consequences, major questions exist related to disparities in disease prevalence, progression, health outcomes, and excessive mortality for many populations, including representatives of some ethnic minority groups. Thus, not only is basic research needed to elucidate our understanding of the mechanisms by which aging is regulated at the cellular level, it is equally important that we involve older Americans—especially women and members of minority populations—in clinical research. As stated by Redmond and Buring, "The unique strength of a well designed and conducted study involving women and minorities is its ability to provide information of direct benefit to these populations, enabling health professionals . . . to make better informed judgements about treatment and care" (Office of Research on Women's Health, 1994).

In light of the close connection between study populations and clinicians' ability to appropriately administer health care to women and men of diverse backgrounds, cultures, and ethnicity across their life span, women and minorities of all ages must be afforded the opportunity to participate in clinical studies. Yet investigators seeking to recruit and retain elderly participants in clinical trials face a number of challenges. Issues of mobility and access to health care, in addition to potentially complex medical problems, for example, can pose particular challenges to investigators seeking to increase older women's participation in clinical research.

The report of an Institute of Medicine (IOM) study commissioned by the National Institute of Health's (NIH) Office of Research on Women's Health (ORWH) to address issues concerning the inclusion of women in clinical trials noted that "There are . . . special considerations for older women related to aging, social roles, and cultural biases. . . . Another consideration is the difference between men and women in the age of onset of disease. Studies of women with heart disease, for example, involve women who are generally 10 to 20 years older than their male peers with heart disease. These older women are often less independent and less mobile. This lack of independence can be a considerable barrier to participation in a study that involves regular visits to a clinical center." The IOM report goes on to state that, "even in an urban area . . . many older women do not have a driver's license or are unwilling to drive into the city . . . . Although concerns about mobility are evidenced in older men and women, the fact that heart disease manifests itself at a later age in women increases the recruitment and retention difficulties inherent in heart disease studies in women" (Stoy, 1994, p. 49).

The IOM report has been helpful to the Office of Research on Women's Health and the NIH as a whole in identifying issues of importance as we work to fulfill the congressional mandate to foster research on women's health issues and seek to promote the inclusion of women of all ages in human subject research. In response to the passage of the NIH Revitalization Act of 1993, the NIH's commitment to require broad inclusion of women and minority members in clinical research was strengthened by Public Law. In a section entitled, "Women and Minorities as Subjects in Clinical Research," the law expanded existing policies for inclusion of women and minorities by requiring:

- that NIH ensure that women and minorities and their subpopulations be included in all human subject research;
- that women and minorities and their subpopulations be included in Phase III clinical trials in numbers adequate to allow for valid analyses of differences in intervention effect;
- that cost is not allowed as an acceptable reason for excluding these groups; and, that NIH initiate programs and support for outreach efforts to recruit and retain women and minorities and their subpopulations as volunteers in clinical studies.

In 1994, the NIH undertook numerous policy and educational activities to ensure that the revised inclusion policies were uniformly implemented across the NIH. The current NIH policy on the inclusion of women in research, "clearly states that women shall be included in clinical studies in numbers proportional to the prevalence among women of the condition under study" (Pinn, 1994, p. iii).

The involvement of communities in research design, implementation, and recruitment is particularly encouraged by the ORWH. The ORWH also convened a meeting to assess the barriers that exist to recruiting and retaining women in clinical studies and has provided researchers with guidance concerning recruitment and retention of women of diverse backgrounds and ages in clinical studies through a published report and outreach notebook produced in collaboration with other entities within the NIH.

In keeping with NIH's commitment to broad inclusion of women and minorities in clinical trials, the ORWH regards as priorities for human subject research those studies that enhance the recruitment of females across the life span as research subjects, especially those groups of women who have been traditionally underrepresented in research. Emphasis is given to addressing the health issues of women of diverse cultures, minority populations, the elderly, rural or inner-city women, as well as those affected by poverty and low socioeconomic status through the fostering and support of research. Special attention is devoted to investigations demonstrating the use of innovative techniques for the successful recruitment and retention of female participants of all ages in research studies, based upon a scientifically appropriate design.

As a result of social and policy changes over the past decade, it is now widely accepted that, in order for the results of research to be widely applicable to the U.S. populace, women and minority volunteers of diverse backgrounds and of appropriate ages of the conditions being studied should be included in clinical research. The ORWH and the NIH as a whole are working to achieve that goal through the uniform implementation of the policies designed to promote both greater equity in research, as well as greater validity, reliability, and medical applicability of research results. The result from such policies that promote equity in participation of research subjects can also serve as the basis for expanded scientific knowledge with broader applicability, and therefore, for better health and health care for women and men of all ages.

In addition, there is a recognition of the need for diversity of those involved in the design, implementation, and interpretation of biomedical and behavioral research, and new programs have been developed and implemented to increase opportunities for women and minorities to enter and advance in biomedical research careers.

REFERENCES

Office of Research on Women's Health (ORWH). (1994). *Recruitment and retention of women in clinical studies* (NIH Publication No. 95-3756). Bethesda, MD: National Institutes of Health.

Pinn, V. W. (1994). Preface. In *Office of Research on Women's Health, Recruitment and retention of women in clinical studies* (NIH Publication No. 95-3756). Bethesda, MD: National Institutes of Health.

Stoy, D. B. (1994). Recruitment and retention of women in clinical studies: Theoretical perspectives and methodological considerations. In *Institute of Medicine, Women and Health Research: Ethical and legal issues of including women in clinical studies* (2 vols.). Washington, DC: National Academy Press.

Offprints. Requests for offprints should be directed to Vivian W. Pinn, MD, Office of Research on Women's Health, National Institutes of Health, 9000 Rockville Pike, Building 1, Room 201, Bethesda, MD 20892.

Journal of Mental Health and Aging, Vol. 6, No. 1, 2000

Contributions of Behavioral and Social Research to Recruitment and Retention of Minority Populations: A Commentary

Norman B. Anderson, PhD

Office of Behavioral and Social Sciences Research
National Institutes of Health, Bethesda, MD

It is a pleasure for me to provide a commentary for this issue on Recruitment and Retention in Minority Populations: Lessons Learned in Conducting Research on Health Promotion and Minority Aging. This issue is the result of research funded under the National Institute on Aging's (NIA) Exploratory Centers for Research on Health Promotion in Minority Populations. I am especially enthusiastic about this issue for two reasons. First, it provides much needed guidance to the scientific community on the recruitment and retention of minority populations for health studies. Second, as a former principal investigator of one the exploratory centers, I am gratified to see the progress and promise of these innovative centers in improving minority health. In this commentary, I would like to briefly describe the mission and responsibilities of the Office of Behavioral and Social Sciences Research (OBSSR) at the National Institutes of Health (NIH) and discuss how the goals of this office relate to issues of recruitment and retention of minority populations in research.

OVERVIEW OF OBSSR

The mission of the National Institutes of Health (NIH) is to fund and conduct research that will improve the health of the public. Congress established the Office of Behavioral and Social Sciences Research (OBSSR) at the NIH to facilitate the growth and development of these important fields. The creation of the OBSSR was in part a recognition that behavioral and social factors are not only significant contributors to health and illness, but frequently interact with biological factors to influence health outcomes. In addition, it was recognized that behavioral and social factors represent important avenues for treatment and prevention.

To further the mission of the NIH, four areas of behavioral and social sciences research must be expanded.

1. We need to identify new behavioral, social risk, and protective factors for disease. Behavioral and social sciences research funded by the NIH has contributed to the discovery of such well-known risk factors as cigarette smoking, high-fat diets, physical inactivity, substance abuse, low socioeconomic status, and many others. Yet, there are unquestionably other behavioral and social potential risk factors for illness that await discovery.
2. We need more research on biological, behavioral, and social interactions as they affect health. It has already been discovered, for example, that psychological stress can impair brain development, elevate blood pressure, suppress immune system functioning, and contribute to coronary occlusion. The hallmark of research on biopsychosocial interactions has been interdisciplinary collaboration, and these efforts must be expanded.
3. We must develop new behavioral and social treatment and prevention approaches. Directing more attention to such approaches will allow us to continue the remarkable progress that has already occurred in the treatment and prevention of an array of disorders such as depression, heart disease, chronic pain, infant mortality, and AIDS.
4. We need more basic behavioral and social sciences research to accelerate advances in such areas as learning and memory, emotion, motivation, perception, cognition, social class, social relations, family processes, and cultural practices. Such research is the foundation for all other behavioral and social sciences research.

Goals of OBSSR

In the OBSSR Strategic Plan, three goals are described which will serve as the foundation of the office's activities for the next 3 to 5 years. These goals are outlined below.

Enhance Behavioral and Social Sciences Research and Training. A major part of the congressional mandate for OBSSR was for it to work to increase support for behavioral and social sciences research and training at NIH, both in the extramural and intramural programs. To accomplish this, OBSSR must assist NIH in identifying and capitalizing on the numerous scientific opportunities that exist in the behavioral and social sciences. These opportunities exist in such areas as the identification of new risk factors; the development of new treatment and prevention approaches; and research on basic behavioral and social processes relevant to health. The office must also work to increase the pool of scientists who are trained to make discoveries in these areas for the ultimate benefit of the public.

Integrate a Biobehavioral, Interdisciplinary Perspective Across NIH. Congress mandated that specific attention be devoted to integrating a biobehavioral perspective into research at NIH. Biobehavioral research, also known as biosocial and biopsychosocial research, combines knowledge and approaches from biomedical, behavioral, and social science disciplines to gain a better understanding of the complex, multifaceted interactions that determine health and pathological human functioning. As such, biobehavioral research represents an exciting new frontier for the health sciences and for NIH. Examples of biobehavioral research include such areas as behavioral cardiology, cognitive and behavioral neuroscience, psychoneuroimmunology, and behavioral genetics.

Improve Communication Among Health Scientists and With the Public. Improved communication among health scientists, and between scientists and the public, is crucial to advancing behavioral and social sciences research and improving health. It was recommended that OBSSR develop a comprehensive communications plan that would involve activities aimed at (1) improving communication and information exchange among behavioral and social scientists; (2) improving communication between sociobehavioral and biomedical scientists; (3) increasing the dissemination of behavioral and social science findings to the public and to health care providers; (4) improving media coverage of behavioral and social sciences research; and (5) ensuring that policymakers are kept abreast of developments in these fields.

The efforts of the NIA-funded Exploratory Centers to improve on the recruitment and retention of minorities in health promotion research, and the resulting research described in this volume, are congruent with the goals of OBSSR. First, these empirically based solutions to minority recruitment and retention are examples of how basic research in the behavioral and social sciences can aid in construction of solutions to scientific problems. That is, without the participation of volunteers in studies funded by the NIH we will be unable to find solutions for some of the vexing health problems facing older minority groups. The behavioral and social sciences are uniquely qualified to identify solutions to this problem, since the issue is indeed one of behavior, occurring with a variety of social contexts. The articles in this issue highlight how a number of methodological approaches—including survey, qualitative, laboratory, and interventional—can be used to identify the social, cultural, behavioral, and psychological predictors of minority participation in research. In addition, the articles demonstrate how the nature of the research itself may serve as a barrier, and how our choice of solutions to the recruitment of minority populations may limit the generalizability of our findings.

The results presented in this issue are also congruent with the OBSSR goal of increasing interdisciplinary research. The Exploratory Centers involve collaborators from such fields as psychology, sociology, anthropology, medicine, social work, epidemiology, health education, biostatistics, and nursing. The complexity of the problem of minority recruitment and retention in health research requires the coalescing of a variety of disciplinary expertise. In fact, one could argue that this type of interdisciplinary effort represents one of the next great frontiers in the health sciences, with the potential to accelerate advances in both basic and clinical research and in public health.

Finally, the research on recruitment by the Exploratory Centers is congruent with the OBSSR goal of greater communication between scientists and the public. Minority communities have frequently been the "objects" of research, with investigators using recruitment strategies that have proven successful with majority populations. The relative failure of this approach has resulted in efforts to gain a better understanding of the perspectives of ethnic minorities concerning the value and nature of health research. Several articles in this issue indeed take a qualitative approach which, rather than constructing a priori hypotheses and procedures, allows minority persons to articulate barriers that might preclude or facilitate their participation in research. This approach not only increases communication between scientists and the communities of interest, but provides valuable information for the design and implementation of health promotion studies.

In conclusion, the issue of recruitment and retention of minority populations for health studies is of critical importance to the overall goal of NIH—to fund and conduct research that advances the understanding, treatment, and prevention of disease. This is especially true given the disproportionate disease burden of ethnic minority populations. Yet, despite the fact that recruitment of minority volunteers has long been recognized as an impediment to finding solutions to minority health concerns, there has been little scientific attention devoted to addressing this issue. This lack of attention is surprising since it is indeed a problem amenable to empirically based solutions. Therefore, I am pleased that the behavioral and social science research community is taking on this challenge, and that the NIA-funded Exploratory Centers are poised to provide empirically based solutions to the problem of minority recruitment and retention in health promotion research.

Acknowledgment. Dr. Anderson will be relocating to the Harvard School of Public Health.

Offprints. Requests for offprints should be directed to Norman B. Anderson, PhD, Harvard School of Public Health, 677 Huntington Avenue, Boston, MA 02115.

Journal of Mental Health and Aging, Vol. 6, No. 1, 2000

The Matching Model of Recruitment

Sue E. Levkoff, ScD
Harvard Medical School, Boston, MA

Becca R. Levy, PhD
Yale University School of Public Health, New Haven, CT

Patricia Flynn Weitzman, PhD
Harvard Medical School, Boston, MA

Existing research on the recruitment of minorities into health research has focused on obstacles present within minority communities and individuals, but has not examined obstacles stemming from research teams and academic institutions. Furthermore, advances in understanding minority recruitment have been limited by a lack of theoretical models to explain recruitment processes. In this article we describe a matching model of recruitment that focuses on barriers and enablers to minority recruitment stemming from both minority communities and research communities. We argue that recruitment success depends on the degree to which there is a collaborative match between the goals of minority communities and research communities. Recognizing and understanding the culture of each community is a prerequisite to a collaborative match. Examples drawn from the recruitment and implementation phases of a cross-cultural study of caregiving are used to illustrate key points.

There is growing recognition among those interested in recruiting participants for health research that the decision making of potential participants has been viewed through a lens that places too little emphasis on social context. Researchers have attempted to analyze how decisions to participate or not participate in research are made by individuals and, in so doing, have utilized decision-making models in which social context is minimized or ignored (Hicks & Lam, in press). While the application of such models may lead to successful strategies for recruiting some middle-class European American research participants, it is likely to fall short when it comes to the recruitment of ethnic minorities (Guo, Levy, Hinton, Weitzman, & Levkoff, this issue; Hicks & Lam, in press; Orono, Koenig, & Davis, 1994). Researchers must now meet federal guidelines regarding the inclusion of minorities in research, but have little empirical information on how social context informs the decision making of minority individuals about research participation, and which recruitment strategies are likely to be effective.

In the field of aging, studies of the recruitment of ethnic minority elders have begun to emerge to fill this research gap (e.g., Picot, Stuckey, Humphrey, Smyth, & Whitehouse, 1996; Young, Edevie, Young, & Peters, 1996; Swanson & Ward, 1995). These studies have been based on the assumption that socially based perceptions of disease influence participation by ethnic minority elders and their family members in health-related research. For example, Picot and associates (1996) outline a model to help researchers understand the cultural meaning of the symptoms of Alzheimer's disease and related dementias (ADRD) among African Americans. They successfully use the model to identify optimal locations and formats for elder recruitment programs. Likewise, Young and colleagues (1996) sought to identify specific barriers to recruitment of African American ADRD caregivers. These researchers found that assigning an African American to the position of recruiter was important, as was addressing caregivers' heightened concerns about privacy and confidentiality.

Although these and other studies have led to improved success in outreach to minority participants, they tend to focus on recruitment exclusively from the point of view of the researcher, such that obstacles to recruitment are viewed as emanating from minority individuals and communities only. Strategies that can be used to overcome recruitment and retention barriers stemming from the social context of the research team and the researchers' home institutions are not delineated. Yet, in our recruitment efforts at the Exploratory Center for Minority Aging and Health Promotion at Harvard Medical School we have found that not only do such barriers exist, but that maximizing minority participation rests as much on addressing research team and institutional barriers as it does on addressing those present within ethnic minority communities themselves. An additional limitation of existing information about recruitment is a lack of theoretical models to aid in the interpretation of recruitment research experiences and to guide subsequent recruitment research (Flores, Castro, & Fernandez-Esquer, 1995).

In this article, we describe a model of ethnic minority recruitment that attempts to balance the perspective of the researchers with that of the potential participants. It is based on researcher experiences recruiting ethnic minority caregivers of elders with dementia into a study examining the impact of culture on how caregivers experience, perceive, and respond to dementia symptoms. The model reported here was formulated after numerous discussions with Exploratory Center researchers and ethnic minority community members about the Center's recruitment failures and successes. Although our study focused on how members of four ethnic groups (African American, Chinese American, Latino, and Irish American) managed Alzheimer's disease, we offer this model to researchers considering the best strategies to recruit ethnic minority individuals into any kind of research.

The general model of recruitment and retention that we propose consists of two different perspectives, and within those perspectives, three different levels. The two perspectives are those of the researchers and those of the ethnic minority groups; each group has its own cognitive and structural style and history. Within both perspectives, three levels are important to recruitment: the macro/institutional level, the mediator/gatekeeper level, and the micro/individual level. Enablers and barriers to recruitment and retention exist within each level. The central tenet of this model is that a match between the perspectives of ethnic minority groups and researchers leads to recruitment and retention success, while a mismatch or conflict between these two perspectives can lead to recruitment and retention failure. An illustration of what is meant by these two perspectives and three levels is found in Table 1. Within the ethnic minority group perspective, community agencies represent the macro level, gatekeepers/health care providers represent the mediator level, and individual participants represent the individual level. It should be noted that the primary access point for gaining participants, for example, the mediator level, may vary. This position could be filled by clergy, social service providers, and so forth, depending upon project goals and target group.

The three-tiered approach applies to the researcher perspective as well and includes academic institutions at the macro level, the research team at the mediator level, and interviewers at the individual level. The contribution of each perspective and level is relevant to recruitment success. Furthermore, levels and perspectives are not separate processes; rather, they dynamically interact. The process by which the three levels and two perspectives interact is mediated at all times by culture in its broadest sense, that is, the institution, researchers, and community members. We define culture as a three-component construct: (1) as a set of local resources available for constructing identity and identifying strategies; (2) as a means for negotiating differences in interpersonal and institutional settings; and, (3) as a form of identity. We will delineate the role of culture in each of the levels in the following description of the levels.

MACRO LEVEL

In assessing the experiences of researchers and potential participants, we found that barriers at the macro level of the participants (Table 2), that is, at community agencies, centered on the fact that service demands were so overwhelming and time constraints so severe, that agency administrators felt they could not participate in the research. To exacerbate the situation, high employee turnover rates at community agencies caused many tentative research collaborations to fall apart. Furthermore, we found that it was important to look closely at the goals and mission of the particular community agency to determine which type of recruiting strategy would likely be most fruitful. Yee (1997) describes several types of community agencies, including monocultural (in which the agency does not acknowledge cultural differences within the workforce or among those served); multicultural (in which the agency explicitly recognizes and appreciates diversity in organizational mission, personnel practices, and service approaches); and sustaining-focus organizations (in which agencies state an explicit mission to serve a specific target group and to meet service gaps for that group). Each agency type varies in the degree to which cultural diversity is emphasized in its

TABLE 1. Overview of the Matching Model of Recruitment

Levels	Ethnic Minority Groups	Researchers
Macro	Community agencies	Academic institutions
Barriers		
Enablers		
Mediator	Gatekeepers/ Health care providers	Research team
Barriers		
Enablers		
Individual	Individual participants/ Caregivers	Interviewers
Barriers		
Enablers		

TABLE 2. Macro-Level Barriers & Enablers to Recruitment

	Ethnic Minority Groups (Community Agencies)	Researchers (Academic Institutions)
Barriers		
	1. Service demands	1. Academic affiliation
	2. Time constraints	2. Tensions between academic centers and local agencies
	3. High turnover rates	3. Academic centers competing to study same groups
Enablers		
	1. Collaboration	1. Offer technical assistance
	2. Mutual gain	2. Recognize local history and cultural beliefs

staffing patterns and community outreach. These differences in cultural emphases manifest in many ways, such as in the types of assurances agency administrators might require from researchers, and how they want their gatekeeper (mediator)-level staff approached.

At the macro level of the researcher, that is, the academic institution, barriers also presented themselves. For example, academic institutions such as Harvard are sometimes perceived of as part of an elite power structure that is not invested in the welfare of the ethnic minority community. Harvard Medical School, located near Roxbury, one of the poorest communities of Boston, has built several new buildings, creating the impression of disproportionate wealth. Boston's Chinatown has experienced considerable tension between major academic centers wishing to expand and local agencies that perceive this as a threat to their patient base. Finally, competition among universities attempting to study the same groups creates confusion for agencies in terms of who is doing what, with whom, and for what purpose. Confusion on the part of community groups about who is doing what can mean that the reputation left behind by a set of researchers from one institution can have fallout (good or bad) when another set of researchers from another institution comes to that community to do research. The end result of this confusion can be a feeling among agency administrators that the benefits of participation in research do not outweigh the costs.

Despite these difficulties, a match in perspectives on the macro level between community agencies and the research team occurred when both groups discussed collaboration. For example, researchers offered a Chinatown community center and a Latino home care agency financial resources and research expertise to develop and implement culturally informed dementia support groups. Agencies received services they needed, and researchers received referrals. Another example of a collaboration that enabled recruitment was when the research team offered technical grant writing assistance to agencies serving Latino and Chinese elders.

Overall, what may be central to recruitment on the macro level is sensitivity on the part of researchers to agency concerns about the commitment of the academic institution to their community. Researchers may need to take on some responsibility as advocates for the community within their home institutions. Also, researchers need to make clear to agency administrators the benefits of participation in the long run, while setting up a collaborative, concrete exchange of services between researchers and administrators that will be beneficial in the short run. An exchange which reflects the unique culture of the community, and how that culture shapes the particular services needed by the community, is most likely to be successful.

MEDIATOR LEVEL

At the mediator level (Table 3), community gatekeepers have the power to give researchers the referrals for recruitment. Barriers can arise when gatekeepers try to "protect" clients. For example, among many Chinese American families, the label of dementia carries a stigma that is perceived as harmful to an entire family. A Chinese American potential participant explained why she refused to participate: "If other people know about this, my grandchildren will have difficulties to get married." In the Chinese community, gatekeepers seemed to try to protect families from social stigma by avoiding officially labeling a client as demented. Many gatekeepers told us that dementia simply does not exist in the Chinese population. Even those who acknowledged the existence of dementia, typically did not encourage families to participate because they believed no treatment to be available and/or saw no real benefit to families for participating. (This dynamic is discussed further by Guo and colleagues in their article in this issue.) The most cooperative gatekeepers were those who identified elders and caregivers who they believed would view research as important. We also found a higher yield of referrals working from the bottom up. That is, we recruited through hands-on service providers who had an intimate knowledge of the elders they serve, rather than dealing with higher level administrators who had little direct contact with families.

From the researcher perspective, barriers and enablers at the mediator level existed within the research team itself. Our research team was made up of people from different academic backgrounds, that is, social gerontologists, medical anthropologists, psychologists, psychiatrists, ethnographers, and health services researchers. These disciplinary differences made collaboration difficult at times, thus impeding recruitment and research processes. For example, an ethnographer initially felt questionnaires were too impersonal and resisted using them in the study. Likewise, some researchers with more quantitative backgrounds failed to appreciate the value of taking field notes and listening to families' candid remarks. Differences in disciplinary perspectives, for example, scientific versus anthropological or quantitative versus qualitative, resulted in pronounced differences in the language used by research team members to describe research experiences and theoretical concepts. The research team was also multicultural, and included individuals with different cultural backgrounds, beliefs, and social histories. These ideological and sociocultural differences created conflicts so contentious that a diversity trainer was enlisted to help the team overcome

TABLE 3. Mediator Level Barriers & Enablers to Recruitment

	Ethnic Minority Groups (Gatekeepers)	Researchers (Research Team)
Barriers		
	1. Protect clients	1. Interdisciplinary differences
	2. Avoid stigma	2. Multicultural differences
	3. Dementia doesn't exist	
	4. No treatment available	
	5. No personal gain	
Enablers		
	1. Readily identify participants	1. Interdisciplinary differences
	2. Believe research is important	2. Multicultural differences
	3. Working from the bottom up	

communication barriers and resolve conflicts. Experiences with the diversity trainer taught researchers that the ideal of diversity is not limited to ethnicity, gender, and sexual orientation, but can apply to academic and professional identities also. Diversity training helped researchers to understand each others' sociocultural language as well as academic language. Above all it taught the research team that, despite differences in language and methodological orientation, there was much agreement across cultures and disciplines represented in the team on the issues in minority health and recruitment that were most important. It was only after the differences were fully discussed that the commonalities could be seen. The experience of working through cultural and ideological differences within the team also helped researchers to work through cultural and ideological differences between themselves and community members. Thus, disciplinary and cultural differences within the research team which began as barriers were transformed, through open discussion and negotiation, into enablers to recruitment.

INDIVIDUAL LEVEL

At the micro/individual level, a number of barriers existed (Table 4). African American caregivers voiced concerns about research due to the legacy of Tuskegee. As one man expressed it, "Any time White people come around asking questions about Blacks, it's usually not for our benefit." Another African American caregiver expressed appreciation of the fact that a researcher was also African American, saying "I don't need another White person coming around to tell me what I should do for my husband." In addition, many caregivers feared stigma to the family, loss of services, or did not trust in the confidentiality of the interviews. This last factor was particularly apparent among Latino participants, some of whom were not citizens, and feared interview information might lead to deportation. Issues of confidentiality were also key for several of the Chinese American caregivers who refused to participate in the study. For example, one Chinese American woman explained: "It is family thing, [we do] not want to talk about it to outsider, please understand." Conversely, all caregivers who agreed to participate expressed that they benefited from sharing their stories and contributing to efforts which might improve the lives of caregivers.

TABLE 4. Micro-Level Barriers & Enablers to Recruitment

	Ethnic Minority Groups (Participants/Caregivers)	Researchers (Interviewers)
Barriers		
	1. Distrust of research	1. Activist agendas
	2. Fear of stigma to family	2. Don't value research
	3. Fear of losing services	
	4. Lack of confidentiality	
Enablers		
	1. Want to share stories	1. Authentic connections
	2. Want to improve the life of others	2. Use of ethnography and qualitative research
	3. Value research	3. Adapt research
		4. Avoid bureaucracy
		5. Rely on existing networks

A barrier at the level of the individual researcher was the fact that some interviewers valued their own activist agendas over the research agenda. Several had been activists in the communities being studied and felt ambivalent about taking on the role of researcher. Some felt that it was unjust to interview caregivers and record their frustrations without, in turn, helping them find solutions. These researchers resisted going on interviews unless they were permitted to work with families on providing social support afterward. Thus, many activist interviewers themselves became like community gatekeepers and raised barriers to recruitment. The team worked through these tensions in several ways. One interviewer found research so intolerable that she left the project. A more successful solution occurred when the research team convinced an activist-oriented researcher that caregivers did indeed benefit from having interested persons listen as they told their stories of caregiving; listening served as a supportive experience to caregivers. (The research team also made many service referrals for participants.) Working through these tensions and retaining the activist-oriented researcher on the team was an enabling factor to recruitment because the activist-researchers' previously established networks allowed us to better map out the local communities of interest.

It is important to include community gatekeepers and elderly individuals in the design and monitoring of the research and in the development of the consent process to ensure that language and content are culturally appropriate. This can be accomplished with a community advisory group which can identify appropriate community members and gatekeepers to participate in research monitoring. Community advisory groups may also make other valuable contributions to recruitment efforts such as helping to identify pools of potential participants, and identifying community needs and cultural factors that may impinge on recruitment success (Parzuchowski, Gelfand, Powell, & Cothorn, 1996). In addition, researchers must continually monitor whether the project is meeting the needs of elderly participants to ensure that the fledgling trust between researchers and elders is maintained throughout the project, and afterward. Trust also allows participants the freedom to express discomfort and withdraw from a research project if necessary.

An additional issue at the micro level has to do with heterogeneity across ethnic minority groups and within groups. For example, the degree of acculturation or assimilation of a given research participant influences who is approached for consent, and how that approach is interpreted. In our study, most of the elderly Chinese Americans recruited as potential participants spoke only Chinese, while in some cases, their American-born sons and daughters spoke English. The English fluency of the U.S.-born children was not always a good indicator of their level of acculturation, however. For example, even though an English-speaking daughter may seem very acculturated in the view of the interviewer, she might follow the Chinese custom of getting her older brother's approval before participating, and require his presence during the interview (a practice consistent with traditional Confucian ethical rules, which confer decision-making authority to an eldest male family member [Elliott, DiMinno, Lam, & Tu, 1996]). Recruiters of ethnic minority participants have to be flexible and adapt the consent process to the particular family dynamic at hand. In one case a Chinese American participant would not give her consent to answer the caregiver survey without first talking to an uncle in California who was the eldest male in her family. Had we not respected her decision, which caused substantial delays in the research process, we would have probably caused her to refuse participation.

Similar family issues emerged during the consent process with African American elders. Whereas consent is typically thought of as provided by one individual, for many African

American participants, family members needed to be involved in the decision to participate, even though only one person ultimately signed the form. In our study, several family members often participated in the interviews with African American caregivers. This may have been a reflection of the distrust that some African Americans have expressed about research. In some cases, it seemed also to stem from contentious family conflicts such that a caregiver's sibling would want to be present because he/she feared the caregiver would give a view of the situation that was biased against him/her.

Additional consent-related barriers at the individual level can arise around language. Although researchers typically attempt to write consent forms in lay language, many are highly technical and difficult to understand without a scientific background or a high level of education. Basic consent forms should use large print and simple language. Local institutional review boards (IRBs) need to encourage simplification of the grammatical structure of consent forms. Other innovative changes, especially for populations with low literacy, include the use of audiotapes, videotapes, or "story book" formats to explain a study or illustrate procedures.

Linguistic matching is also important in the consent process, as well as throughout research. This can be quite expensive to the study. For example, Chinese American participants in our study spoke Cantonese, Toisonese, and Mandarin. This required the study to support a number of researchers who spoke these dialects. The use of interpreters can be aversive to potential research subjects, and connote a half-hearted commitment on the part of the research team to understanding the issues important to the ethnic minority groups being studied. Even when a linguistic match is made between participants and researchers, attention must still be paid to the specific wording used. For example, in our initial consent form, we said "We are talking to immediate family members of older persons with memory problems." This was an issue for the Chinese participants, since married daughters are traditionally considered part of their husband's family, rather than part of their family of origin. Thus, a daughter's involvement in research with her own parents would be an insult to her husband's family. Furthermore, Chinese daughters-in-law often were the de facto caregiver to an ADRD in-law, however, the husband (i.e., the son of the ADRD elder) was viewed as the 'official' caregiver, and needed to both provide consent and be present for the interview. We needed to take these factors into account in the wording of our Chinese American consent form.

It is also critical to understand the specific connotations the same words might have in different ethnic groups. For example, words such as "investigation," "study," and "procedures" appear on all of our consent forms. These words have the potential for bringing up very negative feelings in certain populations. For Chinese American elders who went through the Cultural Revolution, in which they may have been investigated without cause and subjected to harsh interrogations, these words posed a threat. We learned that it was wise not to call ourselves "investigators," but "interviewers." For African Americans, most of whom were familiar with the Tuskegee Study, these words also posed a threat. The word "project" was substituted for "investigation" without changing the meaning of the form. These two examples point to the importance of culturally sensitive language being used in the consent process. Community advisory boards can be very helpful in making the language of consent forms and other instruments culturally appropriate.

Although the consent process highlights many of the barriers we encountered, there were also many successes at the level of the interviewers. Our interviewers established good rapport with the caregivers they interviewed. We believe this was responsible for the high level of retention of our study participants. Another key enabling factor, we believe, was the use of a mix of quantitative research with ethnographic and qualitative research, which allowed us to better understand the varying constructs of dementia held by ethnic minority families.

CONCLUSION

Overall, important lessons about ethnic minority subject recruitment and retention emerged from our experience with this study. We learned that the culture of the researchers, and the institutions they represent, need to be explicitly incorporated into models of recruitment. Barriers within the research team have heretofore not been identified as key to recruitment success; this study demonstrated to us that they can be as important as barriers present in the community. We also found that efforts to create goals common to researchers and ethnic minority groups can result in enhanced participation. Finding ways for mutual gain is important. Equally important is an awareness of local histories between academic institutions and the community, as well as of the local social histories of organizations and the ethnic groups being studied. Community prejudices against an academic institution, while familiar to many of us, have not been commonly included in discussions of recruitment. Furthermore, incorporating key community people into the research team, and establishing or using an existing community advisory group, can aid in recruitment and retention of participants, and in making instruments culturally appropriate. Lastly, we found that the use of qualitative research methods helped to create an environment in which participants, family members, and agency administrators felt comfortable sharing information with us. Good rapport seemed easier to achieve with qualitative interviews probably because they are more naturalistic, that is, more like a real-life conversation, than pencil and paper instruments which can be alienating to participants, especially those who have never before participated in research (Dunigan, 1998). As compared to quantitative methods, qualitative methods can provide more and better opportunities for researchers to convey humane sensitivity to participants, which can help diffuse the distrust felt toward researchers by many minority elders (Morgan & Krueger, 1993). We used qualitative interviews first, and found that the good rapport established during the qualitative interviews carried over into the quantitative assessment. This good rapport also resulted in a high rate of participant retention.

Although recruitment factors highlighted here that reside within ethnic minority communities or individuals themselves have been discussed by others, they have not been balanced with a discussion of factors emanating from academic and research communities. Applying the matching model of recruitment may both enhance recruitment efforts as well as further our theoretical understanding of recruitment and research participation. Wallace (1994) points out that measures of the physical, social, and health service environment are underutilized in individual and population health research. As in recruitment, other levels such as the political/economic environments of the minority community, larger majority community, and the academic institutional community, as well as the public policy environment, may present additional enablers and barriers to success. Continued work using the matching model can help in determining if additional levels are relevant to recruitment success.

REFERENCES

Dunigan, R. (1998, November). *Heterogeneity of caregiving experiences in the African American community.* Paper presented at the annual meeting of the Gerontological Society of America, Philadelphia, PA.

Elliott, K. S., Di Minno, M., Lam, D., & Tu, A. M. (1996). Working with Chinese families in the context of dementia. In G. Yeo and D. Gallagher-Thompson (Eds.), *Ethnicity and the dementias,* (pp. 89-108). Washington, DC: Taylor & Francis.

Flores, E. T., Castro, F. G., & Fernandez-Esquer, M. E. (1995). Social theory, social action, and intervention research: Implications for cancer prevention among Latinos. *Journal of the National Cancer Institute, 18,* 101-108.

Hicks, M., & Lam, M. (in press). Decision-making within the social course of dementia: Accounts by Chinese-American caregivers. *Culture, Medicine, and Psychiatry.*

Morgan, D. L., & Krueger, R. A. (1993). When to use focus groups and why. In D. L. Morgan (Ed.), *Successful focus groups: Advancing the state of the art* (pp. 159-162). Newbury Park, CA: Sage.

Orono, C. J., Koenig, B. A., & Davis, A. J. (1994). Cultural aspects of nondisclosure. *Cambridge Quarterly of Healthcare Ethics, 3,* 338-346.

Parzuchowski, J., Gelfand, D. E., Powell, I., & Cothorn, M. (1996). Recruitment of African Americans to health care research: Lessons from prostate cancer screenings. *Journal of Aging and Ethnicity, 1,* 27-32.

Picot S. F., Stuckey J. C., Humphrey, S. W., Smyth K. A., & Whitehouse, P. J. (1996). Cultural assessments and the recruitment and retention of African-Americans into Alzheimer's Disease research. *Journal of Aging and Ethnicity, 1,* 5-18.

Swanson, G. M., & Ward, A. J. (1995). Recruiting minorities into clinical trials: Toward a participant-friendly system. *Journal of National Cancer Institute, 6,* 1749-1759.

Wallace, R. B. (1994). Assessing the health of individuals and populations in surveys of the elderly: Some concepts and approaches. *The Gerontologist, 34,* 449-453.

Yee, D. (1997) *Organizational contributions to service access and research participation related to older persons of color.* Paper presented at the 1996 meetings of the Gerontological Society of America. Washington, DC.

Young R. F., Edevie S., Young J. H., & Peters, J. (1996). Issues of recruitment and retention in Alzheimer's research among African and White Americans. *Journal of Aging and Ethnicity, 1,* 19-26.

Acknowledgment. Support for this research was provided by the National Institute on Aging and Office of Minority Health of the National Institutes of Health, Grant No. AG 12057. This research was conducted under the auspices of the Exploratory Center for Minority Aging and Health Promotion, supported by the National Institute of Aging (Grant # P20 AG 12057) and the Office for Research on Minority Health of the National Institutes of Health. The authors wish to thank Yeon Chee, Robert Dunigan, Zibin Guo, Ladson Hinton, Humberto Reynoso, Jing Wei, and Donna Yee for their thoughtful contributions to this paper.

Offprints. Requests for offprints should be directed to Sue E. Levkoff, ScD, Division on Aging, Harvard University, 643 Huntington Avenue, Boston, MA 02115.

Journal of Mental Health and Aging, Vol. 6, No. 1, 2000

Recruiting African Americans for Health Studies: Lessons From the Drew-RAND Center on Health and Aging

Stacey Sinclair, PhD
University of Virginia, Charlottesville

Phyllis Hayes-Reams, MD
RAND Corporation, Los Angeles

Hector F. Myers, PhD
UCLA, Charles R. Drew University of Medicine & Science
Los Angeles

Walter Allen, PhD
UCLA, Los Angeles

Jennifer Hawes-Dawson, PhD
RAND Corporation, Los Angeles

Raynard Kington, MD, PhD
RAND Corporation, Los Angeles
National Center for Health Statistics, Hyattsville, MD

African American elderly are underrepresented in health research. This paper highlights recruitment information derived from focus groups with African American elderly conducted through the Drew-RAND Center on Health and Aging. We believe this information can aid in the recruitment and retention of African American elders into health research. Our recommendations include: (1) being sensitive to population concerns, (2) building working relationships with community "gatekeepers," (3) establishing relations with the elderly African American community, (4) being aware of the impact of staff's demographic characteristics on the population, (5) providing transportation, and (6) addressing safety concerns. These procedures enabled us to recruit, and retain, over 5 years, a population of 500 elderly African Americans in Los Angeles.

There is growing recognition of the aging of the U.S. population and the need to effectively address this group's health needs. What is often overlooked, however, is the ethnic composition of the aged and its implications on health care policy. Approximately 13% of the population of the United States, or 31.2 million Americans, are over the age of 65. The percentage of older adults in the United States has increased threefold since 1900 and 22% since 1980 (Ruiz, 1995). However, while previous increases in the proportion of older adults in the population were driven by the number of White elderly, recent expansion of the older adult population is due to the disproportionate increase of older African Americans and other persons of color (Manuel, 1982). For example, between 1970 and 1980 the number of older African Americans increased at a rate of approximately 40% while the number of older White Americans increased at a rate of approximately 25%. Although this trend was temporarily reversed between 1980 and 1990, the rate of increase of African American elderly is expected to exceed that of White Americans into the year 2025.

The problem of the aging population and the changing demographics of this segment of American society is further complicated by marked differences in the functional health status and patterns of morbidity, mortality, and service utilization of older African Americans and White Americans (Bernard, 1993). With a few exceptions African American elderly have a shorter life expectancy, and carry a disproportionate burden of morbidity and mortality from cancer, cardiovascular diseases, diabetes, and other illnesses associated with old age. Older African Americans are also likely to be more functionally disabled and to rate their health as poor than White American elderly (Gibson, 1991; Mendes de Leon et al, 1995; Smith & Kington, 1997).

Despite the growing representation of African Americans among the elderly, and these stable ethnic differences in health risks, morbidity, and mortality, African Americans over the age of 65 are particularly likely to be underrepresented in health surveys and in clinical trials of health interventions (Svensson, 1989). This may lead to a poor understanding of their major health concerns, and the development of health care policies does not address health needs of older African Americans. In an effort to facilitate the recruitment of older African Americans into health research, this article integrates pertinent literature, data from three focus groups with older African Americans, and the experiences of the researchers working with older African Americans at the Drew-RAND Center on Health and Aging to identify recruitment issues that are unique to the population.

RECRUITMENT OF OLDER AFRICAN AMERICANS IN HEALTH RESEARCH

A common reason cited for not including African Americans in health research is that members of this group are difficult to recruit and often fail to complete a study when recruited. Several factors may contribute to these difficulties in the successful recruitment and retention of African Americans in health care research. First, one need only recall the Tuskeegee Study (Jones, 1981) to appreciate the legitimate historical basis for the distrust African Americans have of research (Hornblum, 1998). Second, the reluctance of African Americans to participate in research may have to do with the failure of researchers to consult with community representatives or involve African American collaborators who have the scientific acumen, the community contacts, and credibility to inform the study design. Third, researchers may also fail to establish meaningful, long-term working relationships with key community leaders or community institutions that can serve as conduits for prospective participants, as mediators for the inevitable conflicts that can arise, as well as conduits for dissemination of study findings back to the community (see McNeilly et al., this issue, pp. 91-102). As such, adequate understanding of the distrust that some African Americans feel for the research enterprise may go a long way in ameliorating oft-cited difficulties in obtaining African American research participants.

THE DREW-RAND CENTER ON HEALTH AND AGING

The striking need for more research on the special health and psychosocial needs of African American elderly led to the establishment of the Drew-RAND Center on Health and Aging (DRC) in 1993 at the Charles R. Drew University of Medicine & Science in South Central Los Angeles. This was one of the six Exploratory Centers for Minority Aging & Health Promotion (MAHP) funded by an initiative from the National Institute on Aging (NIA) and the Office of Research on Minority Health (ORMH).

The Drew-RAND Center on Health and Aging (DRC) is a collaboration between Charles R. Drew University, a predominantly ethnic minority academic institution with strong ties to the local African American community in South Central Los Angeles, the RAND Corporation, and a network of senior centers and community-based organizations. The overarching goal of this collaborative effort was the study of health and the aging process in elderly African American residents of inner-city Los Angeles and surrounding neighborhoods. DRC projects addressed several major health issues among older African Americans in the context of an urban community facing a multitude of challenges. In addition to the scientific questions addressed, DRC also implemented a new model of community-based research that builds upon a range of diverse institutions and community groups, all of whom are united by the goal of improving the health and function of elderly urban African Americans.

The DRC focused on several themes, most notably: (1) cooperative research that builds upon the unique contribution of diverse institutions, (2) the development and assessment of measurement tools for use in this population, (3) the assessment of the role of the family in promoting health among older African Americans, (4) the adaptation of previously tested models of health promotion to the unique challenges of this specific community, and (5) the development of new interventions based on a rigorous scientific analysis of newly collected data specific to this community. More specifically, there were four pilot projects conducted by DRC investigators, including: (1) a study of risk factors for stroke in 200 African American elders, (2) a study validating the use of oral and general health assessment instruments in a sample of 100 African Americans elders, (3) a study that assessed gross neurocognitive functioning in 100 African American elders, and (4) a study designed to adapt a two-stage model of community-based screening and geriatric assessment on over 500 African American elders.

The DRC's operation of each of these projects was reviewed by a community advisory board whose members were key stakeholders in the local community, including representatives from senior centers, health centers with geriatric programs, Los Angeles City and County Office of Aging representatives, and older citizens who are active advocates for seniors. In addition, DRC projects included seniors as staff and volunteers who assisted with participant recruitment and in conducting the surveys and assessments.

Our experience at the DRC demonstrated that it is possible to successfully recruit older African Americans to participate in health research. However, successful recruitment of older African Americans into research entails thorough consideration of several factors that may uniquely influence participation. Based on an examination of relevant literature, focus groups with older African Americans about recruitment and implementing the efforts of the DRC, and our experiences at the DRC, we offer several recommendations to other researchers interested in recruiting this population. While these recommendations do not guarantee participation of older African Americans in a given research project, they are offered in an effort to help potential researchers avoid problems that may arise.

FOCUS GROUPS AS A TOOL IN EARLY PLANNING

In order to identify potential obstacles to implementing our projects, we conducted three focus groups with African American elders. The goals for these focus groups were twofold: (1) to identify obstacles to access, and (2) to get the views of potential participants about each of the proposed projects and the initial recruitment plans that were being formulated. We believed that candid feedback from these elderly participants would be important on such matters as how best to advertise the projects, which agencies and individuals would be useful contacts, how best to present the information on the consent form so that African American seniors would be clear about what was being asked of them, and how best to ask the more sensitive questions that were planned in each of the project protocols.

The focus group discussants were contacted through two local senior centers. Groups were run by a moderator and two notetakers, with a DRC representative present. Group meetings were held either at RAND, which is outside the community but afforded the seniors an opportunity to become familiar with this collaborating institution, or at one of the collaborating senior centers in the community. Each focus group lasted approximately 1.5 hours, and all discussants were provided small compensation, transportation and refreshments, and were sent thank-you letters after the meetings were completed.

Each group had between 9 and 13 members. Discussants completed a short questionnaire asking their gender, age, marital status, self-reported health status, and maximum educational attainment. There were slight differences between the three groups, with some groups including more women than the other groups. There was also some variability in SES and in the health and functional status of group members.

A written protocol served as a guide for the discussion, although the leaders sometimes departed from the protocol and discussed issues of concern to discussants that spontaneously emerged during the group. The protocol covered three main areas: (1) discussants' prior contact with research, (2) their reactions to a proposed registry that would provide a pool of subjects from which all current and future projects could recruit, and (3) their feedback on factors that have been identified as potential influences on research participation by this population, such as setting, interviewer characteristics, and contact procedures. Discussants identified a number of key issues and made several recommendations for improving our ability to recruit participants for the various projects. These are summarized below.

Be Specific About the Procedures Used in Your Project

While we should always be specific and clear when explaining a research project for ethical reasons, doing so may be especially important in the recruitment of older African Americans. Specificity and clarity in project descriptions may assist recruitment of older

African Americans because members of this group may be less familiar with the idea of research participation. Most focus group discussants had never participated in any type of research. For example, within all three groups, only 5 discussants had participated in medical research, 3 had participated in commercial research, and 3 to 4 had participated in an interview study conducted by an employee of their senior center. As a result, most did not seem to understand what types of activities actually constitute research. This was revealed when participants gave only examples of medical research in response to a question regarding whether they have ever participated in research. It was not until the focus group moderator specifically mentioned that research can include surveys or interviews that participants acknowledged participation in these types of research projects. Discussants also seemed unclear about the purpose of research, often confusing it with the provision of social services. For example, one discussant mentioned that "many seniors will expect to receive help and advice about their social and physical problems and won't understand why you can't answer their questions or give them what they need if you are a health professional."

Some also expressed reluctance to participate in research using physical measures because they were afraid of being used as "guinea pigs." For example, one discussant said, "I think people are kind of afraid of being guinea pigs. A lot of times when you approach somebody about participating in something like this, they really want to know in detail 'What do you want me to do?'" Other researchers have noted similar suspiciousness regarding health research among African Americans (Mays & Jackson, 1991; Thomas & Quinn, 1991; Williams, 1980). African Americans may be especially suspicious of research because they are aware of past unethical studies using African American participants, such as the Tuskeegee Study. If a particular study does not include physical measures, it may be especially useful to emphasize this with older African American potential participants. Likewise, discussants suggested that taking the time to be especially clear about what will happen in studies using physical measures might help alleviate discomfort with this type of data collection.

Think About How the Project Will Affect the African American Community

Focus group participants also expressed concerns about how the data collected by DRC projects would ultimately be used. These individuals felt that many researchers were not genuinely interested in the issues that affect African Americans and, therefore, would not provide information that was truly beneficial to the community. Although this was not mentioned by our focus group discussants, others contend that African American participants may also be concerned that data collected will be used in a manner that is actually detrimental to them or their community (Thomas & Quinn, 1991). For example, past studies using African Americans have contributed to the perception that they are mentally and physically inferior (Guthrie, 1976; White & Parham, 1990). Such studies have lent "scientific" support to racist policies such as differential sterilization and incarceration (Guthrie, 1976; White & Parham, 1990).

The importance of contending with these concerns is noted by several researchers familiar with conducting research in low-income and/or minority communities (Bengston, Grigsby, Corry, & Hruby, 1977; Josephson, 1970; Milburn, Gary, Booth, & Brown, 1991; Weiss, 1977). They suggest that researchers provide services that are clearly relevant to the target population (e.g., blood pressure screening, talks on pertinent health concerns) and/or emphasize the utility of the data that will be gathered.

Think About How Potential Respondents Will React to the Characteristics of the Project Staff

Some literature also suggests that choosing project staff who are of the same ethnicity as potential participants is an important contributor to successful data collection in minority communities (Jackson, 1991a; Milburn, Gary, Booth, & Brown, 1991; Myers, 1977a; Schwartz, 1970). Our experience with this project also suggests that ethnically matched staff can enhance rapport and other factors conducive to study participation. Providing support for this observation, discussants said that they would be more comfortable with African American staff members than White American staff members. They also pointed out that other characteristics of the staff were equally important. They reported that they would be more likely to cooperate with people who were familiar to them. To this end, they recommended passing out materials describing the DRC and its projects or having the project staff do interactive talks on health issues *before* approaching people about participating in research projects. Discussants also mentioned that they would rather discuss topics, such as health, with other older adults. One such participant stated, "Let's take my daughter. I do not think she has the same feelings that I have about myself. So I would sit down and listen to you [gesturing at another focus group discussant] because I feel like you can relate." Thus, researchers interested in recruiting African American elderly to participate in their studies may be more successful if they include seniors from this community on their research teams. It is important that these seniors be trained to perform meaningful tasks and not just simply be given menial tasks.

Lastly, focus group discussants agreed that the presence of African American principal investigators would greatly encourage them to participate in a research project. In fact, it was implied that the ethnicity of the principal investigators was more important in determining cooperation than the ethnicity of project staff. In addition, they pointed out that competency and politeness of all research staff was paramount for successful recruitment. The following is a typical comment: "We may go to Drew [a hospital staffed largely by African Americans] but if that person does not know what he/she is talking about, we will pick up on it, and after that, anyone you send out we will ignore."

OTHER IMPORTANT LESSONS LEARNED FROM COMMUNITY ACTIVITIES AND THE LITERATURE FORGING EFFECTIVE PARTNERSHIPS FOR RESEARCH

Our recruitment efforts in the community convinced us that conducting community-based research involved establishing effective partnerships with the leaders in community-based organizations and other key "gatekeepers" who were critical to the success of our efforts. (A gatekeeper can be any community-based group or individuals who have access to participants, and whose cooperation and trust must be obtained before approaching potential participants.) Many investigators fail to meet this first requirement by assuming that their study priorities are shared by the community and that their academic and professional credentials are sufficient to give them credibility in the community beyond their home institution. In fact, this attitude can become the greatest obstacle to establishing effective working relationships with the community.

Establishing effective collaborative relationships requires respect for the issues, needs and "turf politics" of the target community. This involves identifying and gaining the trust and support of key community gatekeepers, spending time to get to know them and to be known, seeking their advice, and finding meaningful roles for them to play in the research project. Of particular value is an invitation to serve on a community advisory board as an efficient way of getting their input. Such a group can be very valuable in anticipating problems, suggesting proactive solutions, and opening doors to access participants. This advisory board can also be very helpful to investigators in disseminating study results to the lay community, as well as in helping to identify directions for future research.

CLARIFYING AND RESOLVING CONFLICTS BETWEEN RESEARCH OBJECTIVES AND SERVICE NEEDS

When conducting research in communities with significant needs, investigators whose priority is research alone (rather than research *and* community support) will face a conflict between the need to obtain sound data versus the need to provide services. Many African Americans, including the elderly, are not only skeptical of research itself but also of the techniques of research (e.g., random assignment to treatment conditions, extensive assessments, not immediately intervening to address problems that are mentioned in the interviews). Time, patience, and care must be taken to discuss the tangible benefits to the community (and when those benefits can and will be delivered), and how the benefits hinge on obtaining sound data through reliable research techniques.

GAINING ACCESS TO POTENTIAL PARTICIPANTS

The employment of several types of gatekeepers may be important to the successful recruitment of older African American participants. The insights and endorsements provided by gatekeepers can go a long way in overcoming distrust on the part of potential participants (Becker et al., 1992). In addition, gatekeepers may also be able to assist project staff on issues ranging from publicity to project design (Bengston et al., 1977; Fisher, Auslander, Sussman, Owens, & Jackson-Thompson, 1992; Weiss, 1977).

Collaboration with community gatekeepers, however, may be more difficult and time-consuming than one would assume. Determining which community as well as members to contact requires knowledge of subjective boundaries of your target community, familiarity with local politics and information regarding which individuals, in fact, have contact with members of your target population (Josephson, 1970; Rand & Mebane-Sims, 1992).

Compared to senior centers and nursing homes, the church may be a particularly rich source of older African American potential participants. Older African Americans are reported to depend on the church and fellow church members for support during illness (Johnson & Barer, 1990; Taylor & Chatters, 1986; Walls & Zarit, 1991). It is likely that the same factors that make churches a potentially effective context for health and social services also make them a natural setting for health research. However, it is important to note that accessing subjects through this institution can pose some unique difficulties. According to Gritz and Berman (1992), "the entry phase of church-based network intervention can be time consuming and is unlikely to be cost effective in the short run" because of conflicts between church leaders and health researchers. Time and cost involved in this method of gaining entrance into the African American community may also be exacerbated by the fact that churches also have many levels of gatekeeping (Gritz & Berman, 1992). For example, the pastor may agree to collaborate with a given study but the cooperation of the deacons' board, "nurses" committee, or other groups within the church is usually also required for successful implementation. The current focus groups did not address gatekeepers because we were able to discern relevant gatekeepers through preestablished community contacts. However, focus groups can be helpful in determining who the gatekeepers are, as well as the gatekeeping structure at local institutions and churches, when this information is otherwise unavailable.

SPECIAL NEEDS OF THE TARGET POPULATION

Language

Given that older African Americans may have lower educational attainment and more physical impairments than their White peers, on average, special care may need to be taken to ensure that project materials are clear and easy to read (Becker et al., 1992). When appropriate, participants should also have the option of requesting verbal administration of written materials. However, one must keep in mind that this target population is quite diverse (Jackson, 1988; Manuel, 1982). There is substantial variability in the educational attainment of older African Americans. For example, while approximately one-third (29.2%) of this population has at least received a high school diploma, approximately one-third (32.7%) was not educated beyond elementary school (Ruiz, 1995).

The diversity of this target population was reflected in our focus groups. Although all participants in our three focus groups were recruited from senior centers in the South Central Los Angeles area, they varied in terms of self-reported health, age, and level of educational attainment. Those participants with lower functional competencies were more likely to have difficulties understanding project descriptions, to look to the focus group leaders as sources of medical information, and to have trouble filling out the demographic questionnaire. Even within the "lower functioning" group, variability was such that some participants were able to quickly grasp the project descriptions while others needed much more time and attention.

Extensive open-ended pilot testing is very beneficial in determining the effective wording of forms and measures (Fowler, 1988; Johnson & Cynthia, 1992; Rand & Mebane-Sims, 1992). For example, when developing the National Survey of Black Americans (NSBA), investigators conducted several focus groups to verify and define their concepts with African Americans of different socioeconomic and geographic backgrounds (Jackson, 1991b). Such pilot testing can also help researchers develop solutions for problems associated with recruitment strategies that fail to appreciate the diversity of an older African American sample.

Safety

Potential participants may also have safety concerns that influence their decision to become involved in health research. Despite the low overall rates of crime experienced by older adults in general (Liang & Sengstock, 1981), African American elderly have a greater fear of being victims of crime than older White Americans (McAdoo, 1993). This fear may cause older African Americans to restrict their activities, limit their mobility, and refrain from participating in community events (McAdoo, 1993). This fear may also influence their willingness to participate in health research. Given that such research is likely to involve participants in conversation with strangers, and may be allowing them into their home or in travel to an unfamiliar place, crime stress may interfere with their willingness to participate.

Methods for alleviating this fear may include contacting potential participants by mail or phone before engaging them in person (Carp, 1989), notifying local police stations and churches about the project in order to establish its legitimacy, having a phone number for potential participants with questions to call, or choosing project staff who are known in the community (e.g., other senior residents) (Milburn et al., 1991). When physical exams or other medical procedures are necessary, providing transportation or arranging for the procedures to be conducted in a familiar place may also improve participation rates.

Health

Although it should be obvious, studies of the elderly of all ethnic and socioeconomic groups must include consideration of the functional health status of prospective participants. This includes taking into account limitations in mobility, hearing, vision, and speech. Some investigators exclude persons with these disabilities, which increases internal validity of the findings but at the expense of generalization and external validity of the findings. On the other hand, studies whose goal is to characterize a population will require greater representatives of their sample and, therefore, will have to make provisions for meeting the special needs of those participants with functional impairments (e.g., using protocols with larger type, including staff with sign language capabilities or using hearing-enhancing devices for the hard of hearing, making sure their facility has handicap access).

RECOMMENDATIONS FOR EFFECTIVE RECRUITMENT

A final purpose of the focus groups was to help develop effective and sensitive recruitment strategies for the DRC. The following are some general recommendations derived from relevant literature, the focus groups, and the experiences of researchers at the DRC. It is anticipated that these recommendations are transferable to similar research efforts, though their applicability will be determined by factors unique to a given project.

1. Be sensitive to potential participants' concerns regarding the safety and usefulness of a project. This is likely to be one of the most significant barriers to recruiting participants. In doing so, provide detailed information, handouts and/or have a phone number for participants to call with questions. As will be discussed later, interviewer characteristics and gatekeeper support can be effective in overcoming barriers of trust.
2. Gatekeepers can be instrumental in initiating access to older African American participants. Family, friends, the church, and community leaders may be quite influential with members of this target population who may consider participation in a health study. It is important, therefore, that sufficient time and resources are allocated to establish contact and build working relationships with these key resources. However, also remember that these relationships may be a first step in recruitment efforts. Initial contacts and presentations to these individuals should be as short, engaging, and interactive as possible.
3. Become a familiar face in the target population. Representatives from the DRC learned the importance of this principle early and made special efforts to establish relations with the elderly African American community by giving health talks, speaking with potential participants, as well as developing informational materials stating the accomplishments and goals of the DRC. This familiarity helps to compensate for the distrust engendered by the historical exploitation of minority and/or low-income subjects. Such activities also allow the DRC to repay the community for its cooperation and demonstrate the DRC's interest in and commitment to the concerns of the community.

In the event that establishing such contact and familiarity is not feasible, it can be useful to enlist the help of collaborators who are already familiar to the prospective participants in recruitment efforts (i.e., senior center directors and staff, pastors, community doctors, etc.).

4. Be aware of the potential impact of the staff's demographic characteristics. Our focus groups and literature review support the use of ethnically matched interviewers and examiners whenever possible. Group discussants also expressed greater willingness to talk with other older persons about their health concerns, they also suggested that age and racial characteristics of all personnel may become an issue. Some focus group members emphasized the importance of having African Americans in positions of authority, and all agreed that projects should bring tangible benefits to the community by hiring community interviewers and support staff.
5. Older African Americans are likely to have difficulties with transportation and safety. Therefore, providing transportation, performing exams in locations already frequented by participants, or conducting home exams may be effective facilitators of participation. When travel is required, safe transportation should be provided. In the cases where personal interviews are involved, pre-contact, providing interviewers with identification badges, an information phone number and/or notifying the local police and other community safety officials about the project may serve to reduce fear.
6. Finally, the wording and formatting of advertisements, informational materials, informed consent forms, and instruments should coincide with the abilities and preferences of potential participants. Not attending to these factors may decrease participation and/or increase early drop-out. Pretesting and input from older interviewers can provide insight on the appropriateness of project materials. Despite these precautions, projects may be faced with a particularly heterogeneous group of potential participants, in which case more individualized recruitment efforts will be required.

SUMMARY

Our article describes a successful set of strategies for the recruitment of elderly African Americans to health studies. Over a period of 5 years, the Drew-RAND Center on Health and Aging attracted a population of more than 500 elderly African Americans in Los Angeles to the study. Using procedures described above, we were successful in our efforts to win the confidence of these seniors and to gain their consent to participate in what was expected to become a long-term study of African American health status, experiences, and outcomes under the aegis of the National Institute on Aging Research Center. Unfortunately—due to a combination of factors, many of which the principal investigators could neither anticipate nor control (e.g., recruitment of key personnel to other job opportunities, changing funding priorities)—the Drew-RAND Center on Health and Aging no longer exists.

Given the untimely demise of the Drew-RAND Center, we felt it was necessary to acknowledge the potential ironic consequences of our successful recruitment efforts. In large part, our recruitment efforts were due to our ability to persuade African American seniors, their representatives, and the community gatekeepers that we would be different. Countless times we confronted skepticism and mistrust engendered from a multitude of researchers who had come and gone before us. We countered the frequent comments and expressed belief that, like others before us, DRC would not be around very long. We promised to be a permanent, enduring presence. We made these promises in good faith, based on the expectation that our Exploratory Research Center would evolve into a full-fledged Center and become an established vehicle for research and service among African American elderly in Los Angeles. Since this did not happen, we inadvertently misled those who invested their trust in us.

We cannot help but wonder whether the experiences of DRC will impair the effectiveness of future researchers who approach these same seniors and who endeavor to do research in these same communities (or senior centers). It might also impair these researchers' attempts to call upon the gatekeepers who previously assisted our efforts. We are not sure that the community will find their explanations satisfactory (e.g., elements from the Drew-RAND Center continue as independently funded research projects), that their assurances will be trusted or that they will be able to instill sufficient confidence to ensure future cooperation. For this reason, we caution researchers who hope to change problematic patterns of involvement with neglected or underrepresented populations (e.g., elderly African Americans) to consider how both their presence and their absence will affect future research in the communities they enter.

In summary, the changing composition of the American aging population and the documented differences between Whites and African Americans and other racial/ethnic minority group elders justify the need for more research on these populations, as well as for their inclusion in health studies. While the general consensus is that African American and other minority elderly are difficult to reach and to recruit for participation in health studies, the difficulties many investigators experience may stem from a lack of information and expertise in accessing these populations. The experiences of the investigators and staff of the Drew-RAND Center on Health and Aging demonstrate that African American elderly can be effectively recruited to participate in studies that are viewed as important to the community. Recruitment can be further enhanced if the studies are (1) run by persons who have the trust and respect of community gatekeepers, facilitators, and the elderly themselves, and (2) produce results of both general and specific value to the participants and to the community. We trust that sharing these lessons will prove useful to other investigators who are interested in including elderly African Americans in their research and health studies.

REFERENCES

Becker, D., Hill, D. R., Jackson, J., Levine, D. M., Stillman, F., & Weiss, S. (1992). *Health behavior research in minority populations: Access, design, and implementation* (NIH Publication No. 92-2965). National Institutes of Health.

Bengston, V. L., Grigsby, E., Corry, E. M., & Hruby, M. (1977). Relating academic research to community concerns: A case study in collaborative effort. *Journal of Social Sciences, 33*(4), 75-92.

Bernard, M. A. (1993). The health status of African American elderly. *Journal of the National Medical Association, 85*(7), 521-528.

Carp, F. (1989). Maximizing data quality in community studies of older people. In M. P. Lawton & A. R. Herzog (Eds.), *Special research methods for gerontology* (pp. 93-122). Amityville, NY: Baywood Publishing Co.

Fisher, E., Auslander, W., Sussman, L., Owens, N., & Jackson-Thompson, J. (1992). Community organization and health promotion in minority neighborhoods. In J. Jackson (Ed.), *Health behavior research in minority populations: Access, design, and implementation* (pp. 53-72). Washington, DC: National Institutes of Health.

Fowler, F. (1988). *Survey research methods* (2nd ed., Vol. 1). Newbury Park, CA: Sage Publications.

Gibson, R. C. (1991). Age-by-race differences in the health and functioning of elderly persons. *Journal of Aging & Health, 3,* 335-351.

Gritz, E., & Berman, B. (1992). Recruitment through schools and churches. In J. Jackson (Ed.), *Health behavior research in minority populations: Access, design, and implementation* (pp. 79-89). Washington, DC: National Institutes of Health.

Guthrie, R. (1976). *Even the rat was white.* New York: Harper and Row.

Hornblum, A. M. (1998). *Acres of skin: Human experiments at Holmesburg prison.* New York: Routledge.

Jackson, J. (1988). Survey research on aging Black populations. In J. Jackson (Ed.), *The Black American elderly* (pp. 327-346). New York: Springer Publishing Co.

Jackson, J. (Ed.). (1991a). *Life in Black America.* Newbury Park, CA: Sage Publications.

Jackson, J. (1991b). Methodological approach. In J. Jackson (Ed.), *Life in Black America* (pp. 1-12). Newbury Park, CA: Sage Publications.

Johnson, C., & Barer, B. (1990). Families and networks among older inner-city Blacks. *The Gerontologist, 30*(6), 726-733.

Johnson, C. (1992). Individual recruitment strategies in minority-focused research. In J. Jackson (Ed.), *Health behavior research in minority populations: Access, design, and implementation* (pp. 24-29). Washington, DC: National Institutes of Health.

Jones, J. H. (1981). *Bad blood: The Tuskeegee syphilis experiment.* New York: The Free Press.

Josephson, E. (1970). Resistance to community surveys. *Social Problems,* 117-129.

Kington, R., & Smith, J. (1997). Socioeconomic status and racial and ethnic differences in functional status associated with chronic diseases. *American Journal of Public Health, 87*(5), 805-810.

Liang, J., & Sengstock, M. (1981). The risk of personal victimization among the aged. *Journal of Gerontology, 36,* 463-471.

Manuel, R. C. (Ed.). (1982). *Minority aging: Sociological and social psychological issues.* Westport, CT: Greenwood Press.

Mays, V. M., & Jackson, J. (1991). Aids survey methodology with Black Americans. *Social Science Methodology, 33*(1), 47-54.

McAdoo, J. (1993). Crime stress, self-esteem, and life satisfaction. In J. Jackson, L. Chatters, & R. J. Taylor (Eds.), *Aging in Black America* (pp. 38-48). Newbury Park, CA: Sage Publications.

Mendes de Leon, C. F., Fillenbaum, G. G., Williams, C. S., Brock, D. B., Beckett, L. A., & Berkman, L. F. (1995). Functional disability among elderly Blacks and Whites in two diverse areas: The New Haven and North Carolina EPESE. *American Journal of Public Health, 85,* 994-998.

Milburn, N. G., Gary, L. E., Booth, J. A., & Brown, D. R. (1991). Conducting epidemiologic research in a minority community: Methodological considerations. *Journal of Community Psychology, 19*(1), 3-12.

Myers, V. (1977a). Survey methods for minority populations. *Journal of Social Issues, 33*(4), 11-19.

Rand, C., & Mebane-Sims, I. (1992). Individual recruitment. In J. Jackson (Ed.), *Health behavior research in minority populations: Access, design, and implementation* (pp. 75-78). Washington, DC: National Institutes of Health.

Ruiz, D. (1995). A demographic and epidemiologic profile of the ethnic elderly. In D. Padgett (Ed.), *Handbook of ethnicity, aging and mental health* (pp. 3-21). Westport, CT: Greenwood Press.

Schwartz, D. A. (1970). Coping with field problems of large surveys among the urban poor. *Public Opinion Quarterly, 34,* 267-272.

Smith, J. P., & Kington, R. S. (1997). Race, socioeconomic status and health in late life. In L. G. Martin & B. J. Soldo (Eds.), *Racial and ethnic differences in the health of older Americans* (pp. 106-162). Washington, DC: National Academy Press.

Svensson, C. K. (1989). Representation of American Blacks in clinical trials of new drugs. *Journal of the American Medical Association, 26,* 263-265.

Taylor, R., & Chatters, L. (1986). Church-based informal support among elderly blacks. *The Gerontologist, 26*(6), 637-642.

Thomas, S. B., & Quinn, S. C. (1991). The Tuskeegee syphilis study, 1932 to 1972: Implications for HIV education and AIDS risk education programs in the black community. *Public Health Then and Now, 81*(11), 1498-1505.

Walls, C. T., & Zarit, S. H. (1991). Informal support from Black churches and the well-being of elderly Blacks. *The Gerontologist, 31*(4), 490-495.

Weiss, C. H. (1977). Survey researchers and minority communities. *Journal of Social Issues, 33*(4), 20-35.

White, J., & Parham, T. (1990). *The psychology of Blacks* (2nd ed.). Englewood Cliffs, NJ: Prentice Hall.

Williams, R. (1980). The death of white research in the Black community. In R. Jones (Ed.), *Black psychology* (2nd ed., pp. 403-417). New York: Harper & Row Publishers.

Acknowledgments. This research was conducted under the auspices of the Exploratory Centers for Minority Aging and Health Promotion supported by the National Institute on Aging (Grant No. P20 AG12059) and the Office for Research on Minority Health of the National Institutes of Health. Preparation of this manuscript was also supported by a summer research fellowship from the RAND Corporation to the first author.

Dr. Sinclair was in the Department of Psychology at UCLA, and Dr. Kington was at RAND Corporation when this article was written.

Offprints. Requests for offprints should be directed to Stacey Sinclair, PhD, Department of Psychology, University of Virginia, 102 Gilmer Hall, Charlottesville, VA 22903.

Journal of Mental Health and Aging, Vol. 6, No. 1, 2000

Recruitment of Older African Americans Into Church-Based Exercise Programs

Thomas R. Prohaska, PhD
School of Public Health
University of Illinois at Chicago

Jacqueline Walcott-McQuigg, PhD
College of Nursing
University of Illinois at Chicago

Karen E. Peters, DrPh
Min Li, PhD
School of Public Health
University of Illinois at Chicago

In this study, we identify factors associated with the successful recruitment of older African Americans (age 55+) into a church-based exercise program. Participants who attended the exercise program ($N = 114$) and those who declined (nonparticipants, $N = 55$) were interviewed on measures of health, attitudes, and beliefs about exercise and demographic characteristics. Logistic regression was used to identify differences between groups. Compared to nonparticipants, older adults who participated in the exercise program were more likely to be married, not employed, and to report fewer scheduling conflicts. Nonparticipation was associated with lower self-efficacy for exercise, and a less positive attitude about the benefits of exercise. Participants were more likely to belong to clubs or social groups, and have friends who encouraged them to exercise. However, having friends or family in an exercise group was associated with nonparticipation. Knowledge of these factors may aid in the recruitment of other groups of minority older adults who traditionally have not participated in exercise programs.

In 1993, the University of Illinois at Chicago, School of Public Health, established the Center for Health Interventions With Minority Elderly (CHIME) with funding provided by the National Institute on Aging and the Office for Minority Health. CHIME's work was focused on reducing multiple health risks for minority older adults in different community-based settings. One of CHIME's activities was to investigate factors associated with the recruitment and retention of minority older adults into a variety of community-based health promotion interventions. This paper focuses on factors associated with recruitment of older African Americans into a church-based exercise intervention research study.

Background

Much is known about the health benefits of exercise for older adults, including cardiovascular improvement (Blumenthal et al., 1989), increased muscle strength (Fiatarone et al., 1994), and improved functional abilities (Ettinger et al., 1997). Regular physical activity is also associated with improved mental health, increased self-efficacy, and well-being (Cowper et al., 1991; King, Taylor, & Haskela, 1993; McAuley, Lox, & Duncan, 1993), although findings are not consistent (Blumenthal et al., 1989; Gitlin et al., 1992).

Despite the documented health benefits, most older adults, especially minority older adults, do not participate in regular exercise. According to the Surgeon General's Report on Physical Activity and Health (U.S. Department of Health and Human Services, 1996), fewer than one third of all people age 65 and older report participation in regular, sustained physical activity. In addition, Black, non-Hispanic adults are less likely than White, non-Hispanic adults to participate in most forms of regular physical activity (DHHS, 1996). Given the documented benefits of regular exercise for older adults and the low prevalence of regular exercise in the older population, it becomes important to understand why more older adults, especially minority older adults, do not participate in regular exercise activities.

Reasons for Participation and Nonparticipation

A number of health status and demographic characteristics of older adult populations have been identified as relevant to exercise participation. Using data from the Longitudinal Study on Aging (LSOA), Wolinsky, Stump, and Clark (1995) found that males, younger groups of older adults, those with higher education and those who live alone were more likely to have a regular exercise routine. Similarly, Clark (1999) found that, compared to persons age 70 years and older, persons aged 55 to 69 years were more likely to walk for exercise and to be active in general. Conversely, older females and older persons with poorer self-ratings of health were less likely to exercise (Clark, 1999). Wagner and colleagues (1991) found that older adult members of a health maintenance organization (HMO) who did not participate in a health promotion program were more likely to have lower family income, less formal education, and poorer self-ratings of health compared to older HMO members who did participate. In addition, Morey et al. (1989) compared older veterans who agreed to participate in an exercise program to those who decided not to participate and found that those who refused had more chronic diseases and used more medications than did the exercise participants.

Older adults often cite particular barriers as reasons for not participating in regular exercise. In a study of older adult women, Lee (1993) identified a number of practical barriers to exercise including lack of time, pressure from work and family commitments, poor weather, and inconvenient exercise locations. In addition, there has been research reporting not only on the perceived barriers but also the perceived benefits of exercise. Marcus, Rakowski, and Rossi (1992) adapted a decisional-balance measure which included items on the negative aspects of exercise (barriers) and positive aspects of exercise (benefits) to predict a stage of readiness to participate in regular exercise. This study indicated that persons who were currently exercising were significantly less likely to cite barriers and more likely to agree on the benefits of exercise compared to those who were not currently exercising.

Social support has also been shown to be predictive of exercise behavior initiation and maintenance. Lee (1994) noted that a lack of social support from family was a contributor to nonparticipation in regular exercise activity among older women, and that the influence of social support on exercise behavior decreases with age. In addition, older adults who reported a regular exercise routine were more likely to cite having nonkin social support than those not currently exercising (Wolinsky et al., 1995). On the other hand, some studies have found that social support from family or friends was not significantly associated with older adult participation in exercise.

Finally, an association between self-efficacy and exercise participation has been documented. Specifically, perceptions regarding self-efficacy for performing exercise activities have been found to be positively associated with exercise participation in older adults (Clark, 1995; Sharpe & Connell, 1992). McAuley (1992) noted that perceptions of self-efficacy for exercise were predictive of exercise behavior especially in the early stages of exercise adoption. Furthermore, confidence in one's ability to perform specific exercise activities has been linked to the amount of time per week that an older adult participates in exercise (Clark, 1995). Likewise, self-efficacy in ability to exercise 3 times per week was associated with intention to participate in exercise activities among older adults (Sharpe & Connell, 1992).

Factors Associated With Exercise in Older African Americans

While a variety of factors has been associated with exercise participation in older adults, few investigations have focused on the participation of older African Americans in exercise interventions. Studies that have included sufficient numbers of older African Americans generally find that ethnicity plays no significant role in predicting participation in exercise and physical activity when other psychosocial, health status, exercise beliefs, and demographic characteristics are considered (Clark, 1999; Sharpe & Connell, 1992; Wolinsky et al., 1995).

However, there is some evidence that older African Americans differ in their beliefs and perceptions about exercise. In examining beliefs about exercise and self-reported physical activity among older females, Fitzgerald, Singleton, Neale, Prasad, and Hess (1994), found that African American women were more likely to agree that older people should avoid vigorous exercise and more likely to find it difficult to adhere to a regular program of exercise. The study also found that older African American women were more likely to overestimate the number of days per week and number of minutes per session needed to achieve aerobic fitness. In another study, Airhihenbuwa, Kumanyika, Agure, and Lowe (1995) explored perceptions and beliefs of African Americans toward exercise and found that most considered daily work to be a form of exercise. Specifically, older African American men reported that, after a lifetime of hard physical labor, retirement meant rest rather than leisure time physical activities.

Issues in Recruitment, Participation, and Retention

Unfortunately, most existing research neglects to differentiate between factors leading to participant recruitment and factors associated with adherence or retention in an exercise research program. For example, comparisons between all exercise participants and nonparticipants fail to consider how participation in the exercise program influences perceptions, attitudes, and beliefs. With few exceptions (Marcus, Rossi, Selby, Niaura, & Abrams, 1992; Sharpe & Connell, 1992) previous research typically fails to differentiate between factors leading to exercise participation with changes in attitudes and perceptions that result from participation in the exercise program (i.e., recruitment versus retention). Therefore, in order to understand and improve recruitment procedures, it is necessary to compare participants and nonparticipants before the program has started so that attitudes and beliefs are not confounded by the exercise experience.

In addition, when evaluating factors associated with recruitment, it is important to correctly identify the targeted nonrecruited population. Prohaska (1998) noted that there are legitimate reasons for not participating in exercise and health promotion programs. Among these are lack of exposure to the recruitment message and current participation in other exercise activities. Excluding individuals from the analysis who currently exercise elsewhere allows for a more homogenous group of target individuals in which to study factors concerning recruitment and participation.

For purposes of this study, recruitment was defined as the process wherein someone registered to participate in the exercise research program and appeared on the first day of the intervention when baseline data were collected but no exercise activity took place. Nonrecruited individuals were persons who were exposed to the recruitment message and were not currently exercising elsewhere. This study identifies predictors of successful recruitment of older African Americans into a church-based exercise program. We compare the results of the baseline survey from a group of nonrecruits with a group of individuals who have been successfully recruited but have not yet started the exercise program.

METHODS

Setting

This study was part of a group exercise intervention for older African Americans established in area churches in a large midwestern city. The exercise program targeted parishioners aged 55 years and older in three church settings. Prior to recruitment, key church leaders and active older parishioners were invited to be part of an advisory group and to help plan and implement the exercise research program including participant recruitment. Recruitment procedures were initiated 1 month prior to the exercise program introduction and included weekly announcements in church bulletins and on current-event bulletin boards, public presentations about the exercise program during church services, and an exercise kick-off day that included an information booth and display about the exercise program. Exercise program staff were also available (by phone and in person at the church) to answer questions. Program registration occurred during the church presentation and kick-off, or by phone. The exercise recruitment message and procedures were consistent across churches. The recruitment message stressed that: (1) the exercise program was designed for all older adults including persons who were physically fit as well as individuals with physical difficulties and those who had not exercised in years, (2) the program was free and safe, (3) the exercise classes would be held twice per week in the church during weekday mornings. All recruitment materials were age and culturally appropriate. For example, recruitment flyers included photographs of older African Americans participating in an exercise group and included some persons who were exercising in wheelchairs.

Sample

The sample consisted of two groups of older African Americans from three churches; 123 persons who participated in the church-based exercise program (participants) and 84 persons who did not participate in the exercise program (nonparticipants). All respondents were age 55 years and older. The distribution between participating and nonparticipating respondents was comparable across the three churches. In order to identify the appropriate referent nonparticipant group, nonparticipants who reported that they were not aware of the church-based exercise program and/or were currently participating in another exercise program were excluded from the nonparticipant sample. A total of 27 nonparticipant interviews were excluded as a result of this criterion resulting in a sample of 57 nonparticipants who were aware of the exercise program and who were not currently exercising regularly. Exclusion of respondents with significant missing data resulted in a final sample of 169 (55 nonparticipants and 114 participants).

Assessment Procedures

All interviews were administered face-to-face by a trained research team member. Exercise program participants were interviewed during the first week of the exercise program *prior* to attending an actual exercise class. This allowed for an assessment of perceptions, attitudes, and beliefs about exercise before the development of new attitudes or changes in health status resulting from the exercise experience. Nonparticipants were interviewed *after* the exercise classes began in each of the three churches. All but one of the exercise program participants agreed to be interviewed, and 3 persons who had registered for the exercise program did not attend the first exercise class. The interview lasted approximately 40 minutes. All were paid $5 for their interview. Confidentiality and right of refusal for any questions they did not want to answer was assured before the interview.

Instrument

The survey addressed the five major areas of interest in this study. The instrument included questions about demographics and self-reported health status; barriers to participation in an exercise program; beliefs about the benefits of exercise; support for exercise from family, friends, and doctor; and self-efficacy for participation in an exercise program. Specifically, demographic characteristics included age, gender, marital status (married, not married), employment status (employed full/part-time, not currently employed), religious preference, education, and income. Response options to the income measure were in increments of $5, 000, from less than $5,000 to $25,000 or more. Responses to this question were dichotomized into below $15,000 and $15,000 and higher. Measure of health was based on a single item on self-ratings of health (excellent, good, fair, poor).

Five questions were used to examine the respondents' social support for participating in exercise. Two questions asked if either friends or family encouraged them to exercise. One question asked whether their doctor told them to exercise. Another question asked if their friends and family members exercised regularly. A single question was also included asking if they were a member of a social group or club. All questions were in a yes/no format.

Barriers to exercise participation were measured with a checklist of 12 logistic and motivational barriers associated with nonparticipation with exercise. Respondents were asked "Do any of the following make it difficult for you to exercise?" and a yes/no response was given for each barrier. The seven logistic barriers included transportation, cost, schedule conflicts, no one to exercise with, don't have a good place to exercise and exercise class not available nearby. The six motivational barriers included being too busy, not having enough energy to exercise, fear of exercise outside, fear of injury or pain, and lack of motivation. One additional exercise barrier measure, labeled "any barrier" was created by a dichotomous coding with a 1 when the respondent reported yes to any one or more of the barriers and a 0 when they reported no to all of the barriers on the list.

Self-efficacy was measured with two questions: "What is the highest level of exercise you feel you could participate in?" Response options included Little (sitting, driving, no planned exercise), Mild (standing, walking, bending, reaching, exercise 1 day a week), Active (light physical work, climbing stairs, exercise 2-3 days a week) and Very active (moderate physical work, regular exercise 4 or more days a week). The second self-efficacy item asked the respondent if he or she was confident that they could participate in a moderate exercise program for 45 minutes 2 days per week. Response was in a yes/no format. The two items were combined into a single self-efficacy measure in which respondents who reported yes to the item on perceived confidence and reported that they could be active or very active were coded as 1 on self-efficacy for exercise, and those who said no to the confidence item and/or little or mild on the activity item were coded as 0 on self-efficacy for exercise.

A total of 11 questions was asked about emotional well-being. Respondents were asked to report on a scale from 1 (all of the time) to 5 (never). A factor analysis was conducted with the 11 items which resulted in two factors: a positive emotional well-being factor (Cronbach $\alpha = .60$) and a negative emotional well-being factor ($\alpha = .68$). Positive emotion comprised three emotion items: "How often do you usually look on the bright side of things?" "feel happy?" and "count on good things happening to you?" The negative emotional factor comprised three items: "How often do you get bored?" "feel downhearted and blue?" and "get restless and fidgety?"

Attitudes toward exercise were measured with 15 items. Respondents were asked to report on a scale from 1 (strongly disagree) to 5 (strongly agree) how much they agreed with statements about exercise. A factor analysis was conducted with the 15 items that resulted in two factors; proexercise factor ($\alpha = .73$) and a conexercise factor ($\alpha = .57$). Proexercise comprised seven items: Exercise is fun, important, makes you feel good physically, makes you feel good emotionally, gives a person more energy, improves appearance, and decreases joint pain and stiffness. The conexercise factor consisted of two items; "Exercise is too strenuous" and "I don't like the feelings associated with exercise."

Data Analyses

Bivariate analyses (ANOVA and chi square) were conducted between the nonrecruited and those successfully recruited into the exercise program using participation (participant, nonparticipant) as the dependent variable and individual items from the groups of variables and scales (e.g., demographic characteristics, health status, barriers to exercise, attitudes and belief about exercise, efficacy and social support for exercise, mental/emotional health) as independent measures. Multivariate analyses were then conducted using logistic regression which examined the relationship between participation and independent variables. All demographic characteristics and self-rating of health were entered into the logistic regressions regardless of significance while only significant bivariate associations for all other independent variables were entered into the multivariate analyses. The two measures of attitudes toward exercise (proexercise and conexercise) and the two measures of emotional well-being (positive emotion and negative emotion) were entered into the logistic regression as factors rather than scales. Age was entered into the regression as a continuous measure.

RESULTS

A summary of demographic characteristics of differences between participants and nonparticipants is provided in Table 1. The majority of respondents were female and not currently employed. Age and employment status were the only two demographic measures that differed significantly between the two groups. Compared to nonparticipants, adults recruited into the exercise program were more likely to be older and not currently employed. Self-ratings of health did not differ significantly between the groups.

The most frequently cited barriers to participation in exercise for nonparticipants were schedule conflicts (58.2%), being too busy (36.4%) and lack of motivation (36.4%). The participant group cited having no one to exercise with (32.7%), not having a good place to exercise (23%) and weather (23%) as barriers (Table 2). Compared to those participating into the exercise program, nonparticipants were significantly more likely to report scheduling conflicts, being too busy, and lack of motivation as barriers to exercise participation. The nonparticipant sample was also significantly more likely to report at least one of the barriers listed compared to the participant sample (85.5% versus 65.8%).

Indicators of social support for exercise also differ between participants and nonparticipants. As seen in Table 3, persons successfully recruited into the church exercise program were significantly more likely to be a member of a social group or club (64%). Support for exercise also significantly differed between the two groups with greater encouragement for exercise from friends being given to those recruited into the exercise program (61.4%). Family encouragement for exercise did not differ significantly between the two groups. Contrary to expectation, the nonparticipating group was more likely to say they have friends and family who exercise regularly compared to the participating group (60% vs. 35.1%). A high percentage of both groups reported that, over the past year, their physician suggested that they should exercise (both over 50%). The recommendations to exercise by the physician were significantly more numerous in the participant group (71.1% vs. 54.6%).

TABLE 1. Demographic Characteristics of Recruited and Nonrecruited Exercise Participants

Variable Name	Nonrecruits ($N = 55$) %	Recruits ($N = 114$) %
Age**		
Mean	(65.9)	(69.4)
55-64	45.5	19.3
65-74	45.5	63.2
75+	11.1	17.5
Gender		
Female	83.4	91.2
Male	16.4	8.8
Education		
Less than high school	23.6	34.2
High school	27.3	25.4
College	49.1	40.4
Marital Status		
Married	34.6	41.2
Widowed/never married	65.4	58.8
Income		
Low	36.4	50.9
High	63.6	49.1
Employment***		
Not working	67.3	93.0
Working	33.7	7.0
Self-Rating of Health		
Excellent	20.0	7.9
Good	63.6	71.9
Fair/poor	16.4	20.1

**$p < 0.01$. ***$p < 0.001$.

Differences between participants and nonparticipants on attitudes toward exercise and emotional well-being are presented in Table 4. Attitudes toward exercise differed between the two groups in that recruited exercise participants were more likely to agree with the benefits of exercise (proexercise) (4.28 vs. 4.09) and less likely to agree with the negative consequences of exercise (conexercise) (2.07 vs. 2.27) compared to the nonparticipant group. Emotional well-being also differed between the two groups with recruited exercise participants showing poorer emotional well-being than the nonparticipant group. That is, participants reported that they less frequently experienced positive emotions (2.66 vs. 2.28) and more frequently experienced negative emotions (3.78 vs. 4.15). Finally, self-efficacy (not in table) differed between the two groups with the successfully recruited participants reporting greater self-efficacy for exercise than the nonparticipants (chi square = (1) 12.07, $p < .001$).

Table 5 shows that marital status and employment were significantly associated with participation in the exercise program when combined with the other variables in the logistic regression. The direction of the coefficients shows that being married and not currently employed was associated with exercise program recruitment. Age, which was significant at the bivariate level, is no longer significant at the multivariate level.

TABLE 2. Self-Reported Barriers to Exercise Between Recruited and Nonrecruited Exercise Participants

Barriers to Exercise	Nonrecruits ($N = 55$) %	Recruits ($N = 114$) %
Logistic Barriers		
Transportation	18.2	12.3
Cost	20.0	14.0
Weather	27.3	23.0
Schedule conflicts***	58.2	18.4
No one to exercise with	30.9	32.7
Don't have good place to exercise	18.2	23.0
Exercise class is not available nearby	14.6	22.8
Motivational Barriers		
Too busy***	36.4	6.1
Not enough energy to exercise	21.8	14.3
Fear of exercising outside	10.9	17.5
Fear of injury or pain	9.1	6.2
Lack of motivation*	36.4	20.2
Any Barrier***	85.5	65.8

*$p < 0.05$. ***$p < 0.001$.

TABLE 3. Social Support for Exercise Between Recruited and Nonrecruited Participants

Social Support Variables	Nonrecruits ($N = 55$) %	Recruits ($N = 114$) %
Member of social group or club***	32.7	64.0
Friends/family exercise regularly*	60.0	35.1
Friends encourage you to exercise*	43.6	61.4
Family encourage you to exercise	51.9	66.7
Doctor told you to exercise*	54.6	71.1

*$p < 0.05$. ***$p < 0.001$.

TABLE 4. Composite Psychological Scales of Recruited and Nonrecruited Exercise Participants

Variable Name	Nonrecruits ($N = 55$) %	Recruits ($N = 114$) %	p value
Attitudes toward exercise[a]			
Proexercise	4.09	4.28	.005
Conexercise	2.27	2.07	.042
Emotional Well-Being[b]			
Positive Emotion	2.28	2.66	.008
Negative Emotion	4.15	3.78	.001

[a]Scales range from 1 (strongly disagree) to 5 (strongly agree). [b]Scales range from 1 (all of the time) to 5 (never).

TABLE 5. Logistic Regression Analysis of Recruitment in Exercise Program ($N = 169$)

Variables	Unstandardized Partial Regression Coefficients (b)	p value
Intercept	0.18	ns
Demographics		
Female	1.35	ns
Age	0.02	ns
Education	-0.16	ns
Married	1.73	.02
Employment	-1.95	.03
Income	-0.77	ns
Health status	0.46	ns
Barriers		
Any barrier	-1.22	ns
Schedule conflicts	-2.19	.00
Lack of motivation	-0.92	ns
Too busy	-0.93	ns
Social Support		
Member of social group or club	1.76	.00
Friends and family members in exercise group	-1.83	.00
Friends support me to exercise	1.58	.01
Attitudes		
Proexercise Factor	0.81	.02
Conexercise Factor	-0.27	ns
Emotional Well-Being		
Positive Emotion Factor	1.30	.00
Negative Emotion Factor	-0.28	ns
Self-Efficacy	1.18	.055

Among the barriers to exercise that were significantly associated with recruitment at the bivariate level, only scheduling conflicts remain significant at the multivariate level. Persons with scheduling conflicts are less likely to be in the recruited group. All three social support measures remain significantly associated with recruitment in the logistic regression. The direction of the association remains the same for membership in a social group; having friends' support for exercise being associated with participation, while having more friends and family who exercise, is associated with a lower likelihood of being recruited.

The proexercise attitude measure as well as the positive emotion factor remain significant. Recruited participants are more likely to agree with the positive benefits of exercise and report experiencing positive emotional well-being less frequently than the nonparticipant group. Greater self-efficacy for exercise is associated with recruitment into the exercise program although the significance of the association is marginal ($p = .055$).

DISCUSSION

Findings from this study support the general conclusion that the decision to participate in exercise health promotion research among older African Americans is not random. Many of the factors associated with recruitment found in this study, such as logistical and motivational barriers, social support, self-efficacy and attitudes toward exercise, are similar to those reported for nonminority populations. Demographic characteristics associated with the decision to participate involved differences in marital and employment status. The role of employment status on decisions to participate is consistent with scheduling conflicts, suggesting a general difficulty in setting aside time to participate in a regular exercise routine. These findings are also consistent with Airhihenbuwa and associates (1995) who found that middle-aged and older African Americans felt that their work a sufficient form of exercise. The lack of other demographic variables contributing to decisions to participate may be a result of insufficient power to detect differences or the homogeneity of the sample on some demographic measures.

Although the findings concerning the role of social support on participant recruitment are generally in agreement with expectations, one finding was unexpected. Older African Americans who report they have friends and family in exercise groups were *less* likely to participate in the exercise intervention. It may be that factors contributing to the decisions not to participate in exercise programs with family and friends are also influencing decisions not to participate in our exercise research intervention. Future research should explore the positive and negative influences of having family and friends participating in exercise on one's own exercise behavior.

Finally, the association between emotional well-being and recruitment status was counterintuitive. Older African Americans successfully recruited into the exercise research program reported experiencing less positive emotional well-being than the nonparticipant group. Though prior research has found that older adults currently participating in regular exercise report better emotional health than those not currently exercising, these studies frequently include individuals who have been exercising for some time. With participation in exercise improving emotional well-being in some older individuals (Gitlin et al., 1992), it may be that emotional health is actually lower at the point of being recruited and that for some older African Americans, a reason for participation is to improve emotional health. This finding might also be interpreted as an artifact reflecting the relatively low reliability of the negative emotion scale.

We found 18 persons who reported that they were not aware of the exercise recruitment effort within the church and they were appropriately excluded from the sample. It is possible that they were not exposed to the recruitment message, but it may also be that these individuals were not predisposed or receptive to hear the recruitment message. It may also be that a proportion of these nonparticipants were in the precontemplation stage for exercise behavior. According to Prochaska, DiClemente, and Norcross (1992), persons in this stage process less information about their problem and devote less time and energy to reevaluating themselves.

Our decision to focus our program in the church emerged after attempts to establish it in other community settings. Initial attempts at determining a recruitment setting for the study included senior centers and senior housing. There are many advantages to recruitment of older African Americans in church settings (Ransdell, 1995; Sutherland et al., 1995). Based on data from the National Survey of Black Americans, over 67% of males and 80% of females age 65 to 74 years report church membership (Chatters & Taylor, 1989). Church settings have an existing social support network to facilitate recruitment of potential participants. Church directories and other networking tools such as church bulletins, news letters, and radio service programs provide mechanisms for information dissemination and program awareness (Kumanyika & Charleston, 1992).

However, there are also limitations inherent in recruitment procedures based in church settings, the most important of which is the generalization of the findings. It is not known how frailty and lack of mobility influence church attendance, and how different religious affiliations and religious beliefs influence participation. Future research should determine if there are differential rates of participation in research and health promotion programs based on the recruitment setting (e.g., health care settings, senior centers, churches).

As recommended by Lewis and colleagues (1993), we included recruiters with characteristics similar to the target population, in this case, fellow older parishioners in leadership roles within the church. We followed recommendations concerning active involvement of these community (church) leaders in the development of the recruitment strategy. We concluded that this type of constituency-based model, in which older church members contributed to the recruitment strategy and study design, was a determining factor in recruitment success.

REFERENCES

Airhihenbuwa, C., Kumanyika, S., Agure, T. & Lowe, A. (1995). Perceptions and beliefs about exercise, rest and health among African-Americans. *Journal of Health Promotion, 9*(6), 426-429.

Blumenthal, J., Emery, C., Madden, D., George, L., Coleman, R., Riddle, M., McKee, D., Reasoner, J., & Williams, R. (1989). Cardiovascular and behavioral effects of aerobic exercise training in healthy older men and women. *Journal of Gerontology, 44,* 147-157.

Chatters, L., & Taylor, R. (1989). Age differences in religious participation among Black adults. *Journal of Gerontology Social Sciences, 44,* S183-S189.

Clark, D. (1999). Physical activity and its correlates among urban primary care patients aged 55 years or older. *Journal of Gerontology Social Sciences, 54B,* S41-S48.

Cowper, P., Morey, M., Bearon, L., Sullivan, R., DiPasquale, R., Crowley, G., Monger, M., & Feussner, J. (1991). The impact of supervised exercise on the psychological well-being and health status of older veterans. *The Journal of Applied Gerontology, 10*(4), 469-485.

Ettinger, W., Burns, R., Messier, S., Applegate, W., Rejeski, J., Morgan, T., Shumaker, S., Berry, M., O'Toole, M., Monu, J., & Craven, T. (1997). A randomized trial comparing aerobic exercise with a health education program in older adults with knee osteoarthritis. *Journal of the American Medical Association, 227*(1), 25-31.

Fiatarone, M., O'Neill, E., Ryan, N., Clements, K., Solares, G., Nelson, M., Roberts, S., Kehayias, J., Lipsitz, L., & Evans, W. (1994). Exercise training and nutritional supplementation for physical frailty in very elderly people. *New England Journal of Medicine, 330,* 1769-1775.

Fitzgerald, J., Singleton, S., Neale, A., Prasad, A., & Hess, J. (1994). Activity levels, fitness status, exercise knowledge, and exercise beliefs among healthy, older African American and White women. *Journal of Aging and Health, 6,* 296-313.

Gitlin, L., Lawton, P., Windsor-Landsberg, L., Kleban, M., Sands, L. & Posner, J. (1992). In search of psychological benefits: Exercise in healthy older adults. *Journal of Aging and Health, 4*(2), 174-192.

King, A., Taylor, C., & Haskell, W. (1993). Effects of differing intensities and formats of 12 months of exercise training on psychological outcomes in older adults. *Health Psychology, 12*(4), 292-300.

Kumanyika, S., & Charleston, J. (1992). Lose weight and win: A church based weight loss program for blood pressure control among Black women. *Patient Education and Counseling, 19,* 19-32.

Lee, C. (1993). Factors related to the adoption of exercise among older adults. *Journal of Behavioral Medicine, 16*(3), 323-333.

Lewis, C., Raczynski, J., Heath, G., Levenson, R., Hilyer, J., & Cutter, G. (1993). Promoting physical activity in low-income African-American communities: The PARR project. *Ethnicity & Disease, 3,* 106-118.

Marcus, B. H., Rakowski, W., & Ross, J. S. (1992). Assessing motivational readiness and decision making for exercize. *Health Psychology, 11,* 257-261.

Marcus, B., Rossi, J., Selby, V., Niaura, R., & Abrams, D. (1992). The stages and process of exercise adoption and maintenance in a workplace sample. *Health Psychology, 11,* 368-395.

McAuley, E., Lox, C., & Duncan, T. (1993). Long term maintenance of exercise, self-efficacy, and psychological change in older adults. *Journal of Gerontology, 48*(4), P218-P224.

Morey, M., Cowper, P., Feussner, J., DiPasqual, R., Crowley, G., Kitzman, D., & Sullivan, R. (1989). Evaluation of a supervised exercise program in a geriatric population. *Journal of the American Geriatrics Society, 37,* 348-354.

Prochaska, J., DiClemente, C., & Norcross, J. (1992). In search of how people change: Applications to addictive behaviors. *American Psychologist 47*(9), 102-114.

Prohaska, T. (1998) The research basis for the design and implementation of self-care programs. In M. Ory & G. DeFriese (Eds.), *Self-care and aging.* New York: Springer Publishing Company.

Ransdell, L. (1995). Church-based health promotion: An untapped resource for women 65 and older. American *Journal of Health Promotion, 9,* 333-336.

Sharpe, P., & Connell, C. (1992). Exercise beliefs and behaviors among older employees: A health promotion trial. *The Gerontologist, 32*(4), 444-448.

Sutherland, M., Hale, C., & Harris, G. (1995). Community health promotion: The church as partner. *The Journal of Primary Prevention, 16,* 201-216.

U.S. Department of Health and Human Services. (1996). Physical activity and health: A report of the Surgeon General. Atlanta, GA: U.S. Department of Health and

Wagner, E., Grothus, L., Hecht, J., & LaCroix, A. (1991). Factors associated with participation in a senior health promotion program. *The Gerontologist, 31,* 598-602.

Wolinsky, F., Stump, T., & Clark, D. (1995). Antecedents and consequences of physical activity and exercise among older adults. *The Gerontologist* *35*(4), 451-462.

Acknowledgment. This research was conducted under the auspices of the Exploratory Center for Minority Aging and Health Promotion and supported by the National Institute on Aging (Grant # P20 AG12042) and the Office of Research of Minority Health of the National Institutes of Health.

Offprints. Requests for offprints should be directed to Thomas R. Prohaska, PhD, Community Health Sciences, School of Public Health, University of Illinois at Chicago, 2035 West Taylor Street, Chicago, IL 60612.

Journal of Mental Health and Aging, Vol. 6, No. 1, 2000

Predicting Retention for Older African Americans in a Community Study and a Clinical Study: Does Anything Work?

Shawna V. Hudson, MA
Rutgers, The State University of New Jersey
Piscataway, NJ

Howard Leventhal, PhD
Richard Contrada, PhD
Elaine A. Leventhal, PhD, MD
Susan Brownlee, PhD
Rutgers, The State University of New Jersey
New Brunswick

Recruitment and retention are critical issues for investigators conducting research on elderly and minority populations. Survey data, abetted by observations of our project manager and interviewers, identified factors affecting recruitment and retention in two studies, one community based and the other clinic based. Recruitment differed for gender and marital status by catchment (personal contact versus church or senior centers). Retention was poorer for older persons in the community study but better for the clinic study, replicating existent findings. Retention in the community study was superior for healthier persons, and poorer for those holding self-regulatory beliefs about disease management in the hypertension study. No quantitative measures of social, functional or psychological-affective characteristics predicted retention. Participant comments suggest that accepted methodology is a barrier to retention.

Recruitment and retention are critical issues for investigators conducting research on elderly and minority populations. Herzog and Rodgers (1988) report a linear decline in survey response rates with increasing age showing that the elderly are a difficult group to recruit and retain in studies conducted in community settings. Response rates for the elderly, aged 65 and older, are lower than those for almost all younger age groups. Contrasting results are reported, however, in studies of adherence to medical treatments (Leventhal & Crouch, 1997; Park, Morrell, Frieske, & Kincaid, 1992); adherence is typically higher among patients 65 to 75 years of age than among patients less than 65 years of age or, in some samples, patients over 80 and/or 85 years of age. The community- and clinic-based studies described in this report examine this contrast in African American samples.

In this article we use survey data and the observations of our project managers and interviewers to identify factors affecting recruitment and retention in two studies conducted by the Rutgers University Center for Health Promotion in Elderly African-Americans. The first is a community survey examining the relationships among measures of stress and physical health (community study), the second a survey of clinic patients examining treatment adherence among hypertensives (clinic study). Participants in both studies were informed at the initial point of recruitment that a follow-up interview would be conducted a year later, and intense efforts were made to contact them at the later date. The recruitment sample and the comparison of those completing both baseline and follow-up interviews with those completing only the baseline interview serve as the statistical data for this report.

Preparation for Initiating the Community and Clinic Studies

Three steps were taken to recruit and motivate participation in our studies: examining the catchment, building community support, and hiring visible persons from the local African American community. These steps do not differ widely from those used by other investigators confronting this task for clinical trials (Anderson, Fogler & Dedrick, 1995; Arean & Gallagher-Thompson, 1996; Blumenthal, Sung, Coates, Williams, & Liff, 1995) or programs for health promotion, smoking cessation and exercise (Prohaska, 1997; Wagner, Grothus, Hecht, & LaCroix, 1991).

Examining the Catchment. Our first step was to make sure there was a sufficient minority population in the local area to conduct the proposed studies. County data showed that 29.6% of the 41,711 residents of New Brunswick, NJ, were African American, and 9.3% were over 65 years of age (NJ Legislative District Data Book, 1997). It was clearly feasible to recruit an adequate size sample in the local area. We also took steps to insure that five of the major institutions in the community (Johnson & Johnson Corporation, Rutgers-The State University of New Jersey, Robert Wood Johnson Medical School of the University of Medicine and Dentistry of New Jersey, Robert Wood Johnson University Hospital, and the Middlesex County Health Department) would be supportive of our project. These institutions, along with county and city health agencies, are active promoters of community health programs and employ large numbers of local residents.

Building Support. We next secured the active support of New Brunswick Tomorrow, a community agency sponsored by the Johnson & Johnson Corporation that integrates local business, government, and activist groups in community service. We formed an external advisory board with members from church, activist, and county organizations to obtain their views on project goals. These steps informed community leaders of our study aims and procedures, allowed them to review questionnaires, and gave us valuable feedback on topics and question wording. This enhanced the quality of survey instruments and resolved questions about study objectives and management of privacy.

Personnel. Two steps were taken to insure that respondents would be comfortable with our interviewers. First, we recruited an outreach coordinator who was a 40-year resident of the local community. Her involvement in church and civic activities insured that she was well known and respected by elderly African Americans residents, members of the clergy, and local community leaders. As our coordinator was an early retiree of a New Jersey pharmaceutical corporation, she also was well versed in health issues and health research. Second, we recruited and trained an outstanding group of African American men and women to serve as interviewers. Four were older persons recently laid off due to downsizing by major, national, and regional corporations. Others were graduate and undergraduate students in public health and the social sciences (psychology and sociology).

Theoretical Approach Linking Assessments to Motivation for Participation

As the primary objective of both of our studies was to assess and relate beliefs about health and illness to self-care practices, it was critical that our interviews allowed participants to express their personal beliefs about the factors affecting their health. This objective reflected our self-regulation framework which assumes that personal beliefs play an important role in the selection and maintenance of actions for promoting health and for identifying and treating illness (Leventhal, Leventhal, & Robitaille, 1998; Leventhal, Meyer, & Nerenz, 1980). For example, our self-regulation framework requires that a valid assessment of health risks and self-care will allow individuals to report their own perceptions of the sources of risk, the symptoms or environmental cues indicating the immediate presence of risk, and the methods they believe effective for risk reductions. The questions covered a wide range of factors including lifestyle, stress control, nutrition, exercise, religious values, and so forth. Questions also covered individual's experiences with the health care system, county support agencies, and the stresses of urban living. Thus, the theoretical premises underlying our approach are designed to insure compatibility with our participants' phenomenology and to enhance motivation to participate in follow-up interviews by providing an opportunity to "tell it like it is." For some individuals this was insufficient reason for remaining in the study.

Preparation Specific to Community and Clinic Studies

Community Study: (1) Forging a Link to Participants' Health Interests. Two further steps were taken to enhance personal interest in the substance of the study. First, we conducted four focus groups, two with elderly African American men and two with women, to insure inclusion of issues of interest to our participants and to increase our familiarity with the vocabulary of our cohort. The focus group addressed issues raised by our self-regulation model including perceived causes of threats to health, consequences of health threats, and procedures for prevention. Tape recordings of the focus group proved valuable for generating questions on culturally sensitive topics such as people's experiences of prejudice in the health care system. They also provided the information needed for question wording and the use of scales for closed items. The instruments were further refined in pilot testing and review by our oversight committee.

Second, we anticipated a substantial level of cynicism among residents of our community as their frequent experience with health programs and health surveys rarely preceded observable changes in the delivery of health care. To address how our study would contribute to the delivery of care to elderly African Americans, we indicated that our findings could influence medical education of future practitioners in New Jersey. This possibility was assured as one of our investigators, a professor of medicine at the Robert Wood Johnson School of Medicine, would introduce critical findings into the medical school curriculum.

(2) Newsletter to Sustain Interest and Personal Ties. Every participant was mailed a four-page newsletter twice a year. The newsletter contained three types of information: findings from our study with their implications for improving health practices; results of national studies reporting benefits of diet and exercise for promoting health and the value of screening and medical care for controlling serious chronic illness; and photographs of the interviewers and their backgrounds. This last section emphasized how participation in the study contributed to the progress of the student interviewers, for example, responses to study questions provided data for honors theses and published articles. Progress of the students toward graduation and admission to graduate schools was also reported.

Clinic Study. Steps taken for the clinic study differed from those for the community study as all participants were patients in treatment for high blood pressure at an inner-city clinic staffed by the medical faculty at the Robert Wood Johnson School of Medicine. To insure the interest of clinic staff, initial meetings focused on the factors that our theoretical model indicated to be involved in patients' perceptions of hypertension and their adherence to treatment, for instance, causes of the disease, was it perceived as an acute or chronic condition, the need for medication versus folk remedies, and so forth. Discussions were also held on procedures for identifying and recruiting patients, and the needs for space for interviewing.

Generating Empirical Evidence on Factors Affecting Recruitment and Retention

Although neither of our studies was specifically designed to identify and/or to test hypotheses respecting factors that might affect recruitment and retention, our extensive databases allowed us to examine a wide range of predictors of retention. Our expectation was to replicate findings from prior studies. For example, we expected that completion of the follow-up interviews would be influenced by a person's functional independence (Tennstedt, Dettling, & McKinlay, 1992), age, education, marital status, and income (Psaty et al., 1994).

METHODS

Identifying and Recruiting Potential Participants

Community Study. Limitations of time and funds required a simple and efficient means of identifying participants from among the elderly African American residents in the New Brunswick area. We opted, therefore, for a convenience sample using snowball techniques within four distinctly different catchments: local churches (relationships were established with 12 of the 13 New Brunswick churches with predominantly African American membership), local senior housing units, local senior centers, and community organizations and social service agencies (Civic League of Greater New Brunswick; Middlesex Board of Social Services). Visits to the ministers/directors of these organizations informed them about study aims and secured names of elderly African Americans active in their congregation and/or unit. Our coordinator contacted each of these individuals, described the study aims to them and asked them to supply names of other, potential participants. This procedure generated a list of 334 elderly African Americans, all of whom were residents of New Brunswick, NJ, and adjacent areas (i.e., East Brunswick, Edison, Highland Park, Kendall Park, Piscataway, Somerset, South Brunswick, South River). Recruitment calls to this list yielded a final sample of 187 participants, 37% of whom were reached via personal contacts independent of churches or other organization, 30% of whom were reached through contacts within neighborhood churches, 17% from contacts within senior housing units, 9% through senior citizen centers, and 7% through contacts made at local "health fairs" conducted in conjunction with community agencies. As the number of potential participants varied by site, these percentages do not necessarily reflect the proportion of the elderly African Americans in each catchment.

Clinic Study. The clinic-based sample of 104 individuals in treatment for hypertension was recruited from the roster of patients in treatment at the University Health Center in central New Brunswick. The recruitment process at this site, that is, using clinic records to identify and recruit individuals with diagnosed hypertension, was typical of that used in clinic-based studies. The age range of this sample was younger than the community study and the participants did not overlap.

A list of 232 patients who met criteria for the study was compiled from clinic records. The primary inclusion criteria were: (1) African American by self-identification; (2) aged 45 or older; (3) diagnosed with high blood pressure based on readings of 140/90 mm Hg or higher obtained on three separate occasions; and (4) absent of any conditions that would preclude interview assessment (severe mental illness, dementia, language barriers). To facilitate contact, patients' addresses, telephone numbers, and next scheduled appointments were obtained from their medical records.

Interviewing Procedure

Community Study. The interviewing staff consisted of eight African American interviewers, 5 women and 3 men ranging in age from 21 to 60. All lived in the local area and most were native to Central New Jersey. Each interviewer was assigned a set of participants from our master list, and proceeded to call to arrange a time and place for interviewing, for example, the church, senior center local housing authority, or the participant's home. If participants wished to be interviewed at home but felt uneasy about admitting a stranger into the house, they were called by the outreach coordinator or the neighborhood pastor who served as a reference for the interviewers and the project. Both the baseline and follow-up interviews averaged 90 minutes and were administered approximately a year apart. A $10.00 incentive was offered only for the follow-up interview.

Clinic Study. A $10.00 incentive was given for each of the two interviews: baseline and follow-up. The interviews were conducted by six trained African American interviewers either at the clinic or at a mutually agreed upon alternate location such as the patient's home, church, or senior center. Initial and follow-up interviews took approximately 1 hour and were conducted approximately a year apart.

Clinic participants varied widely in the frequency with which they kept scheduled medical appointments. This required three different procedures for recruitment: scheduling interviews by phone; in-person contact at the scheduled clinic visit if the individual could not be reached by phone; mail and home visit contacts for individuals not reached by phone who did not appear at scheduled clinic appointments.

RESULTS

Recruitment

Community Study. A total of 187 elderly African Americans were recruited from our list of 334 potential participants (Table 1). There were significant differences by gender for each of the different types of recruitment site. The majority of female participants were recruited from senior centers/housing complexes (40%) and churches (34%). By contrast, the majority of men (65%) were recruited by personal contact (gender difference: $\chi^2 = 25.08$, $df = 2$, $p = .0000$). There were significant differences for site of recruitment (personal contact; churches; senior centers/housing complexes) by marital status (married; single widow(er); single never married {$\chi^2 = 18.67$, $df = 4$, $p = .0009$}). The majority of married persons were recruited via personal referral (52%), while over half of the singles (53%) were recruited through senior centers and housing complexes (fewer singles than expected were recruited from churches). Finally, success in recruitment was greater when gender matched. More women recruited through personal referral were successfully recruited by female staff than male staff (85% vs. 15%) and vice versa (64% vs. 36%; $\chi^2 = 27.48$, $df = 1$, $p = .0000$).

Clinic Study. From the original sampling frame of 232 eligible patients, 44% could not be reached by phone, at a clinic visit, or by mail and home visit (Table 1). Of the 139 who were contacted, 106 individuals were recruited. Two patients, however, were unable to finish the interview due to time constraints and illness. Therefore, interview data were collected from 104 subjects, 75% of those contacted.

Retention Community Study

Demographic Factors. A total of 136 of the 187 participants at baseline completed the follow-up interview (73%) (Table 1). Forty (78%) of the 51 noncompleters had withdrawn and 11 (22%) had died. Comparisons of the completers to those who had withdrawn revealed very few differences for any of the basic demographic (age, gender, marital status, education, catchment for recruitment), medical and/or belief measures. The data show that a slightly higher proportion of males than females completed the follow-up (80.8% vs. 69.6%), which is not surprising given that more men were recruited by personal contact and such contact increases follow-up. Those over 80 years of age were less likely to complete the follow-up (61.8%) than those in their seventies (73.6%) or those less than seventy (77.3%).

Medical Factors. The interview covered a large number of factors related to health and use of health care including variables indicative of possible illness (e.g., use of prescription medications, emergency room visits, etc.), preventive behaviors (e.g., physical and dental examination, and screening tests), as well as self-care practices (e.g., exercise), risk behaviors such as smoking, and beliefs in control over health (Table 2a). The completers seemed healthier than the noncompleters, for example, they took fewer prescription medications ($M = 2.31$ vs. $M = 3.18$, $p = .027$), made fewer medical visits ($M = .86$ vs. $M = 1.94$, $p = .037$), had many fewer blood pressure checks in the past year ($M = 5.79$ vs., $M = 11.39$), reported more hours of exercise (e.g., aerobic, $M = .53$ hours vs. $M = .12$; anaerobic, $M = 3.69$ vs. 3.02), and believed it better to treat minor problems, for example, a cold, by themselves (53% vs. 47%) (Table 2a). Only the first two factors, less use of prescription medication and fewer medical visits by those completing the follow-up interview, reached statistical significance in bivariate analyses. No specific factor was significant in a logistic regression model which included prescription and medical visits along with demographic variables of age and gender, though the total model was statistically significant.

Psychosocial Factors. Comparisons of completers and noncompleters yielded no differences of any significant magnitude on a broad range of factors. There were no differences in the social domain, for example, religious attendance, social support, or exposure to life stresses, none in the functional domain, for example, activities of daily

TABLE 1. Demographic Characteristics of the Community and Clinic Participants

	Community Study				Clinic Study			
	Initial Sample Who Completed the Community Study, $N = 187$		Completed One Year Follow-Up, $N = 136$ % Who Completed Follow-Up		Initial Sample Who Completed the Clinic Study, $N = 104$		Completed Follow-Up, $N = 87$ % Who Completed Follow-Up	
	N	%	*N*	%	*N*	%	*N*	%
Gender								
Male	52	27.8	42	80.8	35	33.7	28	80.0
Female	135	72.2	94	69.6	69	66.3	59	85.5
Age								
69 or less	66	35.3	51	77.3	78	75.0	63	80.8
70-79 or less	87	46.5	64	73.6	22	21.2	20	90.9
80 years or older	34	18.2	21	61.8	4	3.8	4	100.0
Marital Status:								
Single	10	5.3	8	80.0	22	21.2	17	77.3
Married	60	32.1	46	76.7	21	20.2	17	81.0
Separated	3	1.6	3	100.0	13	12.5	11	84.6
Divorced	24	12.8	19	79.2	20	19.2	18	90.0
Widowed	90	48.1	60	66.7	27	26.0	23	85.2
Education:								
Less than high school	59	31.6	45	76.3	16	15.4	14	87.5
Some high school	30	16.0	17	56.7	28	26.9	23	82.1
Completed high school	58	31.0	44	75.9	26	25.0	21	80.8
Advanced degree	40	21.3	30	75.0	9	8.7	9	100.0
Recruited through[a]:								
Churches	56	29.9	37	66.1	—	—	—	—
Senior centers/Housing complexes/Health fairs	61	32.6	43	70.5	—	—	—	—
Personal referrals	69	36.9	55	79.7	—	—	—	—

[a]Some participants chose not to provide this information. *N* size differs from that reported in the column head.

TABLE 2a. Medical Information and Health Behaviors of the Community Participants

	Completed the One Year Follow-Up, $N = 136$					Did Not Complete One Year Follow-Up, $N = 51$				
	N	%	*M*	*SD*	Range	*N*	%	*M*	*SD*	Range
Health Care Measures										
Number of prescription medications taken daily*	136		2.31	2.18	0-15	51		3.18	2.82	0-12
Number of medical visits initiated by participants in the past 6 months*	81		.86	1.01	0-6	34		1.94	4.33	0-25
Had blood pressure checked in the last year	136		5.79	6.96	0-48	51		11.39	41.60	0-300
Had dental exams in the last year	70	51.5				19	37.3			
Perceived Control Over Health										
Believe it is better to self-treat minor illnesses rather than see a doctor	86	63.2				24	47.1			

*$p < .05$.

living, reported memory problems, or use of social services, and no differences in the psychological-affective domain, for example, depression, anxiety, stoicism, or experienced stress.

In summary, success in recruitment differed for gender and marital status by catchment; for example, more men and married individuals were recruited by personal contact, and this led to a slightly increased retention rate for men. While two indicators suggested that those remaining in the study were healthier, there were no significant differences between those who completed the follow-up interview and those who did not for any of the social, functional, or psychological-affective measures.

Retention Clinic Study

Repeated efforts to contact participants led to follow-up interviews for 83.7% of the baseline study participants. Only 11.5% withdrew or were unavailable for reinterview. Deaths added an additional 4.8% attrition. As the clinic interview focused on individuals' experiences with their hypertension, it did not include many of the general questions on physical heath, activities of daily living, and psychological health asked of the community participants.

Demographic Factors. Completion rates for the follow-up interview were higher for women (85.5%) than males (80.0%) (Table 1) and participants over 80 years of age (100% vs. 90.9% & 80.8%). These findings were opposite to those of the community study. Completion rates were also low for single participants (77.3% in comparison to all other categories [married = 81.0%; separated, 84.6%; divorced and widowed, 90% & 85%]).

Medical and Self-Regulation Factors. Comparisons of completers and noncompleters yielded no significant differences on any medical factors (Table 2b). The two groups were similar for hypertension status (currently taking medication) and self-regulation beliefs, for example, causes of hypertension (biomedical cause vs. behavioral cause), and belief in their ability to monitor their blood pressure (I can tell when my blood pressure is up). The two groups were also highly similar with regard to their experiences with the health care system (e.g., "My doctor explained [told me] quite a bit about hypertension" [36%] of completers vs. 38% of noncompleters).

Psychosocial Measures. There were no differences between those who did and those who did not complete the follow-up interview on any of the psychosocial measures (Table 3). Those who completed the follow-up and those who did not were similar with regard to their reported level of social support for controlling their hypertension, and similar on religious involvement. Reports of memory problems (i.e., 57% of completers vs. 51% of noncompleters report no problems remembering to take their hypertension medication) and emotional states were also similar. Thus, comparisons between the two groups revealed no medical, social or psychological differences of consequence.

TABLE 2b. Medical Information and Health Behaviors of the Clinic Participants

	Completed the One Year Follow-Up, $N = 87$		Did Not Complete One Year Follow-Up, $N = 17$	
	N	%	*N*	%
Hypertension Status				
Currently taking medication	77	88.5	13	76.5
Belief in Behavioral Causes of Hypertension				
Food and drink contribute to my hypertension[a]	33	37.9	9	52.9
Stress contributes to my hypertension	55	63.2	12	70.5
Personality or temperament contributes to my hypertension	29	33.3	8	47.1
Weight loss contributes to hypertension control	53	60.9	15	88.2
Self-Assessments of Hypertension				
Can tell much of the time when my high blood pressure is up	29	33.3	10	58.8
My own hypertension is very serious[a]	32	36.7	10	58.8

[a]Some participants chose not to provide this information. *N* size differs from that reported in the column head.

TABLE 3. Sources of Social Support and Health Care Experiences of the Clinic Participants

	Completed the One Year Follow-Up, $N = 87$		Did Not Complete One Year Follow-Up, $N = 17$	
	N	%	*N*	%
Religion				
Attends religious services one or more times per week[a]	34	39.0	8	47.0
Strongly believes prayer helps to effectively control own hypertension[a]	56	64.3	14	82.4
Strongly believes prayer helps for own control of hypertension[a]	40	46.0	6	35.3
Social Support				
Strongly believes friends and family help with own control of hypertension[a]	23	26.4	6	35.3
Strongly believes friends and family hinder own control of hypertension[a]	11	12.6	4	23.5

[a] Some participants chose not to provide this information. *N* size differs from that reported in the column head.

DISCUSSION

Three aspects of the empirical analysis merit attention. First, as one might expect, retention was higher among the clinic sample (83.6%) than the community sample (72.7%): this difference is largely unchanged when mortality is taken into account (87% vs. 77%). Although the level of education was somewhat higher for participants retained in the clinic sample, it is a younger group with many more of its members in the work force lacking medical health coverage. Their lack of coverage and their desire to recount their experiences with barriers to seeking treatment for their hypertension may account for why a larger proportion of this group, in contrast with the community sample, were motivated to participate in the follow-up interview.

The second point of interest is the different relationship between demographic factors of age and gender to follow-up in the two studies: men and younger persons were more likely to complete the follow-up interview in the community sample, and women and older persons were more likely to complete the follow-up in the clinic sample. With the exception of the unexpectedly high rate of retention of men in the community study, the findings are in accord with published data; older persons are less likely to be retained in survey studies (Herzog & Rodgers, 1988), and older persons are more likely to be adherent to treatment for hypertension (Park et al., 1992).

Third, in both samples medical factors and/or self-regulatory beliefs appeared to be impediments to follow-up. Failure to follow-up was higher in the community sample for individuals on multiple prescribed medications and heavier users of medical care. Although the small sample size of the clinic sample precluded statistical significance, self-regulatory beliefs associated with failure to follow up replicated prior findings. For example, failure to follow up was more frequent for those who believed they could feel changes, that is, monitor changes in their blood pressure, and attributed their pressure to lifestyle rather than biological factors, for example, personality, stress, and weight (Meyer, Leventhal, & Gutmann, 1985). Apart from these effects, however, it is the absence of differences across a broad range of social, functional, and psychological measures that stands out. Questionnaire items designed to assess function, psychological status, and so forth, do not predict sample maintenance.

Qualitative responses provided by study participants identified other methodological factors that created barriers to continued participation in both the community and clinic studies. These included interview length and the use of scales rather than open-ended questions. For example, participants in the community study often remarked that, "I began to get tired. The first 30 minutes are alright. Then after that, it is like talking to a pole . . . I have to be doing something and sitting here doing this, it annoys me." Others said, "some of the scales are kind of confusing," "some of the questions sound like they're repeating in a different way," and "some of these scales are not in jive with what you're asking . . . strongly agree, disagree. A lot of people get that twisted in their minds and can't answer properly." We concur with critics who argue that the methodological constraints set by current research practices fail to take account of cultural differences and create barriers to sustained participation (Rogler, 1999). Indeed, we believe that the psychometric requirement to use multiple items to assess a small number of variables results in underspecified models, less thoughtful responses by participants, and reduced quality of research. Moreover, we believe these effects hold for nonminority as well as minority populations.

Our use of multiple, interpersonal strategies to compensate for these problems of length and repetition was not in vain. The majority of the participants in both studies consented to do the follow-up interview regardless of the methodological inconvenience involved. They did so because, in the words of one participant, "I hope that it will do some good. . . . It [the data] needs to reach people who need to know about these things." In addition, participants wanted "some of the things we're doing and saying here to help other people." Because our theoretical and research approaches took these concerns into account by employing staff members from the community who were well known and respected, showing that the data were being used by students and other members of the research team, and enhancing the visibility of the project and its connection to community organizations, we were able to reduce the tendency of participants to view the community and clinic studies as examples of elite institutions needlessly exploiting people's time. We conclude that these efforts, in the absence of convincing quantitative findings, influenced immensely our retention rates.

REFERENCES

Anderson, L. A., Fogler, J., & Dedrick, R. F. (1995). Recruiting from the community: Lessons learned from the diabetes care for older adults project. *The Gerontologist, 35*(3), 395-401.

Arean, P., & Gallagher-Thompson, D. (1996). Issues and recommendations for the recruitment and retention of older ethnic minority adults into clinical research. *Journal of Consulting and Clinical Psychology, 64*(1), 875-880.

Blumenthal, D., Sung, J., Coates, R., Williams, J., & Liff, J. (1995, April). Recruitment and retention of subjects for a longitudinal cancer prevention study in an inner-city Black community. *Health Services Research, 30,* 197-205.

Bureau of Government Research. (1997). *New Jersey Legislative District Data Book* [17th District Page]. New Brunswick, NJ: Rutgers, The State University of New Jersey.

Herzog, A. R., & Rodgers, W. L. (1988). Age and response rates to interview sample surveys. *Journal of Gerontology: Social Sciences, 43*(6), S200-S205.

Leventhal, E. A., Leventhal, H., & Robitaille, C. (1998). Enhancing self-care research: Exploring the theoretical underpinnings of self-care. In M. Ory & G. DeFriese (Eds.), *Self-care in later life* (pp. 118-141). New York: Springer Publishing Co.

Leventhal, E. A., & Crouch, M. (1997). Are there differences in perceptions of illness across the lifespan? In K. J. Petrie & J. A. Weinman (Eds.), *Perceptions of health & illness: Current research and applications* (pp. 77-102). The Netherlands: Harwood Academic Publishers.

Leventhal, H., Meyer, D., & Nerenz, D. (1980). The common sense representation of illness danger. In S. Rachman (Ed.), *Contributions to medical psychology* (vol. II, pp. 7-30). New York: Pergamon Press.

Meyer, D., Leventhal, H., & Gutmann, M. (1985). Common-sense models of illness: The example of hypertension. *Health Psychology, 4,* 115-135.

Park, D., Morrell, R., Frieske, D., & Kincaid, D. (1992). Medication adherence behaviors in older adults: Effects of external cognitive supports. *Psychology and Aging, 7,* 252-256.

Prohaska, T. (1997). The research basis for the design and implementation of self-care programs. In M. G. Ory & G. H. DeFriese (Eds.), *Self-care in later life: Research, program and policy issues* (pp. 62-84). New York: Springer Publishing Co.

Psaty, B. M., Cheadle, A., Koepsell, T. D., Diehr, P., Wickizer, T., Curry, S., Von Korff, M., Perrin, E. B., Pearson, D. C., & Wagner, E. H. (1994). Race- and ethnicity-specific characteristics of participants lost to follow-up in a telephone cohort. *American Journal of Epidemiology, 140*(2), 161-171.

Rogler, L. H. (1999). Methodological sources of cultural insensitivity in mental health research. *American Psychologist, 54,* 424-433.

Tennstedt, S. L., Dettling, U., & McKinlay, J. B. (1992). Refusal rates in a longitudinal study of older people: Implications for field methods. *Journal of Gerontology: Social Sciences, 47*(6), S313-S318.

Wagner, E., Grothus, L., Hecht, J., & LaCroix, A. (1991). Factors associated with participation in a senior health promotion program. *The Gerontologist, 31,* 598-602.

Acknowledgments. This research was supported by the National Institute on Aging, Minority Aging and Health Promotion Exploratory Center Grant AG12072, by a National Institute on Aging Minority Graduate Research Assistant Supplement P20 AG12072, and by the Rutgers University Institute for Health, Health Care Policy, and Aging Research. The authors give special thanks to Brenda Sadler for her invaluable input.

Offprints. Requests for offprints should be directed to Shawna Hudson, MA, Department of Sociology, Rutgers, The State University of New Jersey, 54 Joyce Kilmer Avenue, Piscataway, NJ 08854-8045.

Journal of Mental Health and Aging, Vol. 6, No. 1, 2000

Health Promotion Research With Mexican American Elders: Matching Approaches to Settings at the Mediator- and Micro-Levels of Recruitment

Helen P. Hazuda, PhD
Meghan Gerety, MD
John W. Williams, Jr., MD, MHS
Valerie Lawrence, MD
Walter Calmbach, MD
Cynthia Mulrow, MD
University of Texas Health Science Center
San Antonio, TX

Minority elders are inadequately represented in health promotion research. A contributing factor may be that recruitment approaches have not been well adapted to the life experiences of these populations. This article examines recruitment approaches used in several health promotion projects with Mexican American and European American elders, using the Matching Model of Recruitment as a theoretical framework. According to the model, matches between the perspectives of ethnic minority groups and researchers lead to recruitment and retention success, while mismatches or conflicts lead to failure. The article highlights how researchers in four small projects conducted by the Hispanic Healthy Aging Center adapted their recruitment approaches to match the perspectives of gatekeepers at the mediator level and individual participants at the micro level of recruitment, as defined by the Matching Model. Factors contributing to successful recruitment and retention are summarized and rated in terms of their relative importance for both groups of elders, and for clinic and community settings.

Inclusion of ethnic minority elderly in health promotion research is of critical concern. As the U.S. elderly population grows, it is becoming more racially and ethnically diverse (U.S. Bureau of the Census, 1992). The proportion of European Americans will decrease from 87% of the elderly population in 1990 to 65% in 2050. At the same time, that of African Americans will increase from 8.0% to 12.0% of the elderly population; of American Indians from 0.4% to 0.8%; and of Asian/Pacific Islanders from 1.4% to 8.2%. Hispanic Americans, the most rapidly growing segment of the U.S. elderly population, will increase more than fourfold from 3.7% to 15.3% of the elderly population. The majority of Hispanic elderly will be Mexican Americans. While their numbers are rising, ethnic minority elderly, particularly African and Mexican Americans, have a higher prevalence of chronic conditions and disabilities than do European Americans (Clark & Gibson, 1997; Hazuda & Espino, 1997). However, older adults generally, and ethnic minority elderly in particular are inadequately represented in clinical and health promotion research (Arean & Gallagner-Thompson, 1996; Carter, Edward, Malmgren, Martin, & Larson, 1991; Lovato, Hill, Hertert, Hunninghake, & Probsfield, 1997). An important contributing factor may be researchers' lack of awareness of the need to adapt recruitment strategies for these populations (Arean et al., 1996; G. Marin & B. Marin, 1991; Swanson & Ward, 1995).

The Hispanic Healthy Aging Center (HHAC) at the University of Texas Health Science Center at San Antonio was one of six Exploratory Centers for Minority Aging and Health Promotion funded by the National Institute on Aging and the Office of Minority Health. The HHAC conducted four small pilot projects as a prelude to designing culturally appropriate interventions to promote independent function in Mexican American (MA) and European American (EA) elderly. In this article, we describe the goals, target population, study design, and subject burden for each project, along with the recruitment and retention approaches used. Adaptation of approaches to different study settings is highlighted.

To provide a theoretical framework for examining these approaches, we used the Matching Model of Recruitment (Levkoff, Levy, & Weitzman, this issue). The model is based on the premise that the decision-making process leading individuals to participate or refuse participation in research is influenced by the social context of potential participants and their community agencies, as well as that of the researchers and their home institutions. As shown in Table 1, the model includes two perspectives, operating at three levels. Perspectives of the ethnic minority groups and the researchers are based on their own cultural and structural styles and history, and influence interactions at the macro/institutional level, the mediator/gatekeeper level, and the micro/individual level. The model's central tenet is that matches between the perspectives of ethnic minority groups and researchers across levels lead to recruitment and retention success, while mismatches or conflicts between these perspectives at any level can lead to recruitment and retention failure. The focus here is on matches at the mediator- and microlevels of the model.

TABLE 1. Components of the Harvard Matching Model of Recruitment

	Perspective	
	Ethnic Minority Group	Researchers
I. Macro	Community Agencies	Academic Institutions
II. Mediator	Gatekeepers/Health Care Providers	Research Team
III. Individual	Individual Participants/Caregivers	Interviewers

Project 1: Determinants of Exercise in the Elderly

The goal of this project was to obtain information for designing an office-based physician intervention to increase physical activity in MA and EA elderly. The target population was MA and EA patients of primary care physicians. The study was cross-sectional. Subjects were asked to complete a single assessment administered in their homes, lasting approximately 3 hours which included both self-report and performance measures of physical function.

Initial recruitment success centered on mediator-level (gatekeeper) variables. First, in order to sample the target population, we had to gain the cooperation of primary care physicians for patient referrals. This was relatively easy because of an existing collaboration between the HHAC and the South Texas Ambulatory Research Network (STARNET) which comprised physicians in private practice who had worked with us in the past. STARNET staff randomly selected subjects from the pool of eligible MA and EA patients presenting for medical care and made the initial contact to explain the study during their office visit. Individuals who agreed to participate were then referred to HHAC staff who contacted them by telephone to arrange the home interview. Thus, the active cooperation of STARNET staff was critical to recruitment success.

We also had to develop and maintain strong liaisons with STARNET office staff responsible for selecting and referring patients to assure their continuing commitment to the study. Because an HHAC research associate had been meeting with office staff twice monthly for an extended period before the study began, open communication was already established. When the HHAC study began, this research associate worked with the STARNET office staff to train them to perform the random selection and referral process. The associate continued to meet with them on a monthly basis. We believe a key to recruitment success was constant contact with office staff, and an awareness of special concerns and needs of different sets of STARNET staff. Each office was unique. For example, in some offices the staff really enjoyed being treated to special foods. Others appreciated a small monetary "thank you." And still others preferred office presentations about the study results and their impact on patients.

An additional component of the Project 1 Exercise Study was the establishment of focus groups to obtain qualitative information about cultural variation in the meaning of physical activity. Four focus groups were planned for the MA and EA groups, organized by age and physical activity level. Focus group participants were drawn from those individuals who had completed the home interview. Although all 8 focus groups were completed, recruitment was difficult for several reasons. First, the pool of eligible subjects for each group was greatly restricted because of strict inclusion criteria. Second, groups were conducted in a central location, but geographic distance still presented barriers. Third, the length of the initial interview (3 hours) discouraged some potential participants from getting involved in this additional phase of the study. Fourth, no monetary incentives were provided.

Project 2: Functional Recovery After Elective Major Surgery

The goal of Project 2 was to examine the natural history of postsurgical recovery to identify precursors of successful, protracted, or limited recovery; and to identify potential intervention points. The target population was MA and EA elders undergoing major elective abdominal surgery. The study design was longitudinal and involved high subject burden. Subjects had to complete six assessments over a 6-month period. Each assessment was 1-2 hours long and included self-report and performance measures of physical function, as well as open-ended questions about coping strategies.

Subjects were recruited from surgical units at two university-affiliated teaching hospitals and private hospitals in the community. The major recruitment challenge at the mediator-level was gaining access to adequate numbers of MA and EA subjects within these settings. Because the project principal investigator (PI) had attending privileges at both teaching hospitals, we had access to surgery schedules (once the hospitals' Institutional Review Boards approved the study). However, to gain support from surgeons responsible for the care of potential study subjects, the PI "advertised" the study at a UT Medical School conference. Letters were also written to senior surgery faculty asking them to ask their residents to encourage patients to participate. HHAC research associates made daily contact with the general surgical services and operating room schedulers at each hospital to identify patients scheduled for surgery and to prescreen for eligibility. The research associates then contacted the patient directly and performed the preoperative assessment in patients' homes.

To access patients in the private hospitals, the PI had to establish a cooperative relationship with a number of private surgeons. This was done by adapting our outreach program to the surgeons' tightly scheduled days. Communication about the study was limited to two to three sentences, and a protocol was established that did not require the surgeon to put in any effort. At any given time, approximately 20 to 24 private surgeons were involved in the study. Research associates contacted the surgeon's office staff twice weekly to obtain referrals. Developing and maintaining the office staff's interest in the study was difficult because there was little or no face-to-face contact. A $5 per patient referral fee provided some incentive. Nonetheless, because offices did not provide the study with the actual surgical schedule for all their patients, there was no way of knowing what proportion of eligible patients were actually referred to the study.

At the microlevel, a major challenge was convincing patients about to undergo major surgery to enroll in a study requiring multiple interviews over the coming 6-month period. Five research associates were needed to work on subject recruitment at this level. Four of the five were MA, and one was EA. Research associates placed heavy emphasis on rapport building. Their goal was to treat subjects informally, like friends, rather than more formally, as research subjects. Overall, 64% of eligible patients agreed to enroll, with virtually identical response rates among MAs and EAs (64% and 63%, respectively). There were no significant differences in overall enrollment rates based on the research associates' gender or ethnic background. However, a male research associate had a significantly higher response rate among men than women (71% vs. 25%, respectively; $p < 0.05$), regardless of the subject's ethnic background.

Three general strategies were used to retain subjects throughout the 6-month study period. First, follow-up interviews were conducted at the participant's home to ease the burden. Second, "thank you" cards were sent immediately following each visit, and a reminder was attached indicating the date of the next visit and total number of visits remaining. Third, at each visit research associates focused on maintaining rapport and reinforcing the importance of the study for helping others undergoing similar surgery. Nonetheless, response rates in both ethnic groups drifted down over time, suggesting that additional strategies were needed (see Table 2). Only 62% of MA elders and 48%

of EA elders completed all follow-up assessments. Follow-up response rates were significantly higher among MA elders than EA elders for completion of all six assessments. Follow-up rates were similar for the five research associates, and no significant differences were observed based on the research associates' gender or ethnic background, or hospital setting.

Project 3: Impact of Depression on Physical Function

The goal of this project was to obtain information to design interventions for depression to be delivered in primary care settings, and to lessen the impact of depression on physical function. The target population was patients attending primary care clinics. The design was longitudinal, and involved moderate to high subject burden. Subjects were asked to complete a baseline interview of 1-2 hours which included a comprehensive assessment of depression, as well as self-report and performance measures of physical function. Twenty-minute telephone follow-up interviews were done 4 times over the next year. Participants were offered $5.00 for each interview.

Subjects were recruited from primary care clinics at two university-affiliated teaching hospitals, and a community primary care clinic located in a lower socioeconomic status (SES), predominantly MA neighborhood. As with the two previous projects, a key element to successful recruitment at the mediator-level was gaining access to patients at each site. The PI was a primary care physician with attending privileges at the two university-affiliated hospitals. He gave special presentations to his colleagues at these hospitals to convince them of the study's importance and to assure them that it would have a minimal impact on their normal clinic routine. To gain access to patients at the community clinic, the PI built on the university's established role in training minority physicians who later practiced in the community. Several of the physicians at the community clinic had done their residency with him, and were familiar with clinical research. For these reasons, most were enthusiastic about having their patients participate in the study. These feelings were reinforced by periodic educational programs which the PI provided to both the physicians and their community advisory boards.

To minimize the burden on physicians and their staffs, HHAC research associates recruited subjects directly in the clinic waiting areas. Willing participants were taken to a clinic exam room to give informed consent and complete an initial 5-15-minute

TABLE 2. Ethnic Group Distribution and Follow-Up Response Rates for Project 2

Time points	MA		EA		*P*-value ethnic differences
	N	(%)	*N*	(%)	
Pre-operative	128	(100)	134	(100)	—
Post-operative					
1 week	116	(1)	110	(82)	0.028
3 weeks	118	(92)	107	(80)	0.004
6 weeks	109	(85)	112	(84)	0.726
3 months	100	(78)	92	(69)	0.083
6 months	104	(81)	92	(69)	0.019
Completed all	79	(62)	64	(48)	0.023

screening interview. To assure that patients would not miss their appointments and the physician's practice would not be delayed, a brightly colored tag was placed on the patient's chart indicating that the patient was being interviewed for a research study, giving the location, and noting that the interview could be interrupted if the physician was ready to see the patient. Because this approach required cooperation from clinic personnel responsible for patient flow, HHAC research associates nurtured positive relationships with the staff. For example, researchers were careful not to disrupt clinic activities. They also brought special foods, arranged celebrations for the staff on holidays such as Valentine's Day or Halloween, and joined in office parties. Updates of research progress and findings were given to the staff regularly.

At the micro level of recruitment, key concerns were the study topic (i.e., mental well-being), the length of follow-up, and the ability to track low SES, primary care patients over this time period. Research associates had to establish trust with the participants at the initial screening and subsequent baseline interview in order to lay the groundwork for later telephone assessments. This was accomplished by emphasizing confidentiality, and behaving in ways that demonstrated the researchers' sensitivity to the patients' cultural background. It was important that research associates were bilingual and bicultural, familiar with the San Antonio community, and able to accommodate Spanish-speaking MAs (29% Spanish speakers). Some modification of inclusion criteria and patient incentives was also required. Initially, research associates had difficulty contacting patients by telephone to complete follow-up interviews. Therefore, inclusion criteria were changed to require that subjects have telephones and a stable home address. The telephone number of a relative or close friend who would be able to contact the subject for the study, if needed, was also obtained, and the reimbursement for completed interviews was increased from $5.00 to $10.00.

Among the 228 subjects who met screening criteria, 218 (96%) agreed to enroll in the study and complete the baseline assessment. Among the entire sample, participation rates were similar among MA and EA elders, and exceeded 80% at each follow-up. In addition, 76% of MA and 69% of EA elders completed all four follow-up assessments. Response rates among older subjects tended to be higher than those among younger subjects, regardless of ethnic group (see Table 3).

Three MA research associates were responsible for recruiting patients and completing the assessments. For the most part, effective approaches to recruitment and retention were similar for MA and EA elders, but some differences were observed. Among EA elders, matching the research associate and participant on gender and ethnic group did not seem to matter. Among low-SES MA elders, however, gender matching was often helpful. This was particularly true for married women whose husbands served as family gatekeepers. For example, low-SES MA husbands would often refuse to allow a male research associate to speak with their wives, but when recontacted by a female research associate would allow the wife to participate in the interview. Adult children also seemed to serve as gatekeepers for their elderly parents more often among MA than EA elderly. Among MA elders generally, it was important to realize that decisions to participate in a research study were often family decisions, and that interaction with the entire family group, not just the individual subject, was required.

TABLE 3. Follow-Up Rates by Ethnic and Age Group

	Younger & Older Subjects Combined			Younger (18-59 Years Old)		Older (60 + Years Old)			
	Mexican American *N* (rate)	European American *N* (rate)	*p* Value Ethnic Differences	Mexican American *N* (rate)	European American *N* (rate)	Mexican American *N* (rate)	European American *N* (rate)	Total *N* (rate)	*p* Value Subgroup Differences
Baseline	157	61		109	25	48	36	218	
3-month	150 (96%)	56 (92%)	.232	102 (94%)	20 (80%)	48 (100%)	36 (100%)	206 (95%)	.033
6-month	139 (89%)	56 (92%)	.626	95 (87%)	23 (92%)	44 (92%)	33 (92%)	195 (89%)	.611
9-month	141 (90%)	54 (89%)	.808	96 (88%)	21 (84%)	46 (96%)	33 (92%)	196 (90%)	.363
12-month	136 (87%)	49 (80%)	.293	93 (85%)	19 (76%)	43 (90%)	32 (89%)	187 (86%)	.352
Completed all	120 (76%)	42 (69%)	.300	80 (73%)	13 (52%)	40 (83%)	29 (81%)	162 (74%)	.070

Project 4: Adaptation to Subclinical Disability in Mexican American Elders

Project 4 (the Adapt project) focused on the functional stage of subclinical disability—a stage in which the elderly maintain independence in basic and instrumental activities of daily living even though they have functional limitations (i.e., restrictions in performing fundamental physical and mental actions). The project had three goals: (1) to develop a typology of adaptive strategies used by MA elders to maintain independence in everyday living, (2) to obtain the information to design interventions to promote independence in MA elders with subclinical disability, and (3) to develop an instrument to detect and quantify subclinical disability in MA elders. The target population for goals 1 and 2 was community-dwelling MA men and women. The target population for goal 3 included an EA comparison group representing a comparable range of physical function and SES. The study design was cross-sectional and involved low-to-moderate participant burden. Subjects for goals 1 and 2 were asked to complete a one-time assessment that included self-report and performance measures of physical function, and a 2-3-hour qualitative interview exploring adaptive strategies. Subjects for goal 3 were asked to complete a 1-hour assessment that included self-report and performance measures, and a 45-minute quantitative instrument, developed from the qualitative data, to detect and quantify subclinical disability.

Several recruitment options were considered for both parts of the study. Option 1 was to identify senior centers or churches that served MA and EA elderly from a broad range of SES backgrounds. Option 2 was to select a random sample of MA and EA elderly from census tracts within different SES areas. Option 3 was to "piggyback" onto an ongoing study that included MAs and EAs from diverse SES backgrounds. The third option was clearly the best in terms of time, labor intensity, and costs of recruitment, but required access to subjects in an appropriately designed ongoing study. If such a study could be identified, the key recruitment challenge at the mediator level would be gaining the cooperation of study investigators and staff.

The PI for the Adapt project was able to identify a study to piggyback onto, that is, the San Antonio Longitudinal Study of Aging (SALSA). Because the Adapt PI had established a collaborative relationship with the SALSA PI in several previous studies, gaining initial agreement to piggyback was easy. However, a number of mediator-level issues arose during the actual conduct of the project. For the SALSA PI and staff, the top priority was maximizing participation in SALSA and doing nothing to jeopardize future follow-ups. For the Adapt PI and staff, the top priority was completing their own study on a timely basis. When conflicts arose, SALSA staff, who functioned as gatekeepers for Adapt participants, put SALSA priorities first.

Recruiting subjects (n = 24) for the goal 1 and 2 qualitative interviews went very smoothly. The senior SALSA research nurse (an older bilingual-bicultural EA female, fluent in Spanish) knew the participants well. For each gender and SES stratum, she easily identified subjects across a range of physical function who had already completed SALSA, were articulate enough in Spanish or English to respond to qualitative questions, and who would be willing to complete the interview. She made the initial contact with prospective interviewees and prepared them for subsequent contact by the HHAC research associate. Because of the research nurse's introduction and rapport with participants, the Adapt research associate was able to recruit and interview participants much more easily than might otherwise have been the case.

Obtaining the subjects ($n = 400$) needed for the goal 3 study involved more complex gatekeeping. The piggyback protocol required that potential participants complete SALSA before enrolling in Adapt. Participant burden was minimal since assessments common to both studies were administered only once. The referral process was as follows. A list of participants who agreed to be contacted was drawn up every week, cross-checked to verify they met certain criteria, and e-mailed to the Adapt research associate. Occasionally, SALSA demands were so heavy that the research nurse was unable to make the list without jeopardizing SALSA, and there was a gap of 2 or 3 weeks between lists. Nonetheless, the process generally went smoothly until the final 6 months, when SALSA recruitment was slowing down and available subjects often did not meet the criteria for Adapt participation. Additional time was needed to handle this, but the result was that 90% of SALSA subjects referred completed the Adapt.

Because of the way the Adapt was piggybacked, many micro-level recruitment issues were addressed in SALSA. Four elements contributed to successful recruitment and retention across ethnic groups and neighborhoods: (1) assembling the appropriate staff, (2) forming liaisons with key individuals and agencies within and/or serving the MA community, (3) identifying specific barriers to recruitment and retention within each type of neighborhood and implementing specific strategies to overcome them, and (4) identifying and utilizing specific facilitators of recruitment and retention within each type of neighborhood. Appropriate staff had to have several qualities. First, they needed cultural sensitivity; that is, they must be able to accommodate differences between their own view of the world, and that of the MA and EA subgroups in each socioculturally distinct neighborhood. Second, they had to have formal and informal skills in both Spanish and English to accommodate MA Spanish speakers. Third, they had to be knowledgeable about the historical experiences of diverse MA and EA subgroups within the community. Fourth, they had to have perseverance, that is, be willing to stay with the subjects, making repeated contacts over an extended period of time, if necessary, to enlist their participation.

DISCUSSION

This article describes recruitment approaches from several health promotion projects in terms of matches at the mediator and micro levels defined by the Matching Model of Recruitment. Table 4 lists a number of general factors included in these approaches and rates their relative importance for success in recruiting MA and EA elders from clinic and community settings.

To a large extent, factors contributing to recruitment success were the same in both settings and ethnic groups. The greatest difference between settings occurred at the mediator level, reflecting the pivotal role of collaborating physicians and their staff as gatekeepers for clinic populations. Had the community study utilized senior centers, churches, or other community agencies as the source of its subject population, mediator-level differences across settings would have been reduced further.

The greatest difference between MA and EA groups occurred at the micro level, and reflected cultural differences in language usage and the role of family members in an individual's decision to participate in health research projects. For some MA participants, it was necessary to conduct the interview and to interact with them in Spanish.

TABLE 4. Factors Contributing to Recruitment and Retention Success for Mexican American and European American Older Adults

Factor	Clinical Setting		Community Setting	
Mediator Level				
Tier I: Collaborators (e.g., physicians, PIs, community centers)	MA	EA	MA	EA
1. Pre-established relationships with potential collaborators.	**	**	**	**
2. Match approach to the culture of targeted collaborators.	***	***		
3. Design research activities to have negligible impact on regular office routine or conduct of collaborating studies.	***	***	***	***
4. Provide outreach training and/or educational programs for collaborators.	*	*		
5. Give regular updates on research progress and results.	**	**	**	**
Tier II: Collaborators' staff				
1. Adapt research activities to normal clinic routine and staff priorities.	***	***	***	***
2. Tailor reinforcements to staff culture of each office (e.g., special snacks or food, money contributions to office party pool, participation in staff social events, regular updates of research progress of results, monetary incentive for individual staff referrals, etc).	***	***	***	***
3. Demonstrate sensitivity and concern for referred individuals.	***	***	***	***
Individual Level				
Tier I: Family members of participants				
1. Build rapport and interact with family members as joint decision makers.	**	*	**	*
2. Accommodate Spanish-speaking family members.	**		**	
3. Adapt approach to married female participants to meet husband's preferences (e.g., secure husband's approval for wife's participation, use female interviewers).	**		**	
4. Accommodate care-taking responsibilities for grandchildren.	**		**	

TABLE 4. ***(Continued)***

Tier II: Individual participants	MA	EA	MA	EA
1. Emphasize importance of study and reinforce elders' strong sense of altruism.	**	**	**	**
2. Emphasize confidentiality, especially for sensitive topics (e.g., mental well-being).	**	**	**	**
3. Demonstrate familiarity with the community and sensitivity to participant's cultural background.	***	***	***	***
4. Modify approach to match the world-view and life context of diverse population subgroups.	***	***	***	***
5. Accommodate Spanish speakers.	***		***	
6. Conduct follow-up interviews at home or by telephone.	**	**	**	**
7. Send Thank You cards and reminders.	**	**	**	**
8. Provide continued encouragement at follow-up visits.	***	***	***	***
9. Provide monetary incentives for completed assessments.	**	**	**	**

Importance to recruitment retention success: * = Somewhat important; ** = Very important; *** = Essential.

The former required that all research instruments undergo cross-cultural adaptation. This is a labor-intensive process that involved not only translation from English to Spanish, but adaptation to the idiom, daily context, and lifestyle of traditional MA culture. The importance of family decision making and husbands' influence on wives' participation among MAs has been noted by others (Naranjo et al., 1998). Some have suggested that same-ethnicity interviewers enhance rapport with Hispanic subjects (Marin & Dirksen, 1991). However, we found no evidence in either ethnic group that matching interviewers and subjects on ethnic background affected participation. On the other hand, gender matching increased response rates among both MA and EA women in the surgery study, and among MA women in the depression study. The most important characteristics of good recruiters and interviewers, however, regardless of their ethnic group or gender, were sensitivity to the participants' cultural background and the ability to adapt approaches to match the world view and life context of individuals from diverse population subgroups. This is precisely what would be predicted on the basis of the Matching Model of Recruitment.

REFERENCES

Arean, P. A., & Gallagher-Thompson, D. (1996). Issues and recommendations for the recruitment and retention of older ethnic minority adults into clinical research. *Journal of Consulting and Clinical Psychology, 64*(5), 875-880.

Carter, W. B., Elward, K., Malmgren, J., Martin, M. L., & Larson, E. (1991). Participation of older adults in health programs and research: A Critical review of the literature. *The Gerontologist, 31*(5), 584-592.

Clark, D. O., & Gibson, R. C. (1997). Race, age, chronic disease and disability. In K. S. Markides & M. R. Miranda (Eds.), Minorities, aging, and health (pp. 107-122). Thousand Oaks, CA: Sage Publications.

Hazuda, H. P., & Espino, D. V. (1997). Aging, chronic disease, and physical disability in Hispanic elderly. In K. S. Markides & M. R. Miranda (Eds.), *Minorities, aging, and health* (pp. 127-148). Thousand Oaks, CA: Sage Publications, Inc.

Levkoff, S. E., Levy, B. R., & Weitzman, P. F. (2000). The Matching model of recruitment. *Journal of Mental Health and Aging, 6,* 29-38.

Lovato, L. C., Hill, K., Hertert, S., Hunninghake, D. B., & Probstfield, J. L. (1997). Recruitment for controlled clinical trials: Literature summary and annotated bibliography. *Controlled Clinical Trials, 18,* 328-357.

Marin, G., & Marin, B. (1991). *Research with Hispanic populations* (23 ed.). Newbury Park: Sage Publications.

Nagi, S. Z. (1979). The concept and measurement of disability. In E. D. Berkowitz (Ed.), *Disability policies and government programs* (pp. 1-15). New York: Praeger.

Naranjo, L. E., & Dirksen, S. R. (1998). The recruitment and participation of Hispanic women in nursing research: A learning process. *Public Health Nursing, 15*(1), 25-29.

Swanson, G. M., & Ward, A. J. (1995). Recruiting minorities into clinical trials: Toward a participant-friendly system. *Journal of the National Cancer Institute, 87*(23), 1747-1759.

U.S. Bureau of the Census. (1992). Sixty-five plus in America (Current Population Reports, Special Studies, P-23). Washington, DC: U.S. Department of Commerce, Bureau of the Census.

Acknowledgment. This research was conducted under the auspices of the Exploratory Centers for Minority Aging and Health Promotion and supported by the National Institute on Aging (Grant # P20 AG12044) and the Office for Research on Minority Health of the National Institutes of Health.

Offprints. Requests for offptints should be directed to Helen P. Hazuda, PhD, Department of Medicine, University of Texas Health Science Center at San Antonio, San Antonio, TX.

Journal of Mental Health and Aging, Vol. 6, No. 1, 2000

Minority Populations and Psychophysiologic Research: Challenges in Trust Building and Recruitment

Maya McNeilly, PhD
Duke University Medical Center, Durham, NC

Marc Musick, PhD
University of Texas at Austin

Jaye R. Efland, BS, Jannie T. Baughman
Paul S. Toth, PAC, Terry D. Saulter, BS
Lekeisha Sumner, BS, Andrew Sherwood, PhD
Duke University Medical Center, Durham, NC

Patricia Flynn Weitzman, PhD
Sue E. Levkoff, ScD
Harvard University Medical School, Boston, MA

Redford B. Williams, Jr., MD
Duke University Medical Center, Durham, NC

Norman B. Anderson, PhD
Office of Behavioral and Social Sciences Research
National Institutes of Health, Bethesda, MD

Minority populations have been historically underrepresented in scientific research. Various factors have been cited to account for this. In this article we focus on overcoming this barrier of distrust of the medical system which can influence the participation of older African Americans in research. We outline four types of trust that we found essential to successful recruitment. We also present the relative effectiveness of various methods used to recruit older African Americans. Our hope is that the discussion of some of the challenges and presentation of strategies used to overcome these challenges will be helpful to investigators attempting to conduct research with minority populations.

Various factors have been cited to explain the underrepresentation of minority group members in clinical research. A notable factor for African Americans, in particular, may be the Tuskegee Syphilis Study of the 1930s in which treatment was withheld from African American men (Thomas & Quinn, 1991). Older African Americans may be especially distrustful of the medical system because they were alive during the Tuskegee debacle, and/or because many feel they have been subjected to a high degree of abuse in the American medical system (Brawley & Tejeda, 1995). Racism and abuse present in medical and other institutions have created in many African Americans a sense of fatalism (Brawley & Tejeda, 1995). This fatalism manifests itself in the belief that there is little reason to seek medical help or participate in a clinical trial (Ad Hoc Committee on Cancer in the Poor, 1990). Unfortunately, even for those who try to obtain medical care, obstacles related to cost, transportation, and lost wages can stymie their efforts (el-Sadr & Capps, 1992; Levkoff, Levy, & Weitzman, in press). These same practical obstacles can interfere with the successful recruitment of minorities.

Of course, not all obstacles to the recruitment of African American and other minority individuals into clinical research stem from minority groups themselves. For example, only recently has there been a mandate on the federal level to include minorities in clinical trials (National Institutes of Health, 1994). Up to this point researchers may have been dismayed over the poor representation of minorities in clinical trials, but did not feel compelled to overcome recruitment barriers. The NIH mandate has changed that. Levkoff, Levy, and Weitzman (2000) discuss other barriers to minority participation created by researchers. For example, building trust with gatekeepers and community leaders can be particularly important because these individuals are considered trustworthy and credible by their constituents, that is, potential participants. If gatekeepers and community leaders trust in the intentions of the researchers and the benefits of the research, they are likely to become powerful partners in the recruitment process. One way researchers can effectively forge trustful relationships with gatekeepers is by involving them in all stages of program development (Lenfant, 1995), and offering tangible services and assistance back to them in return for their recruitment help (Levkoff et al., 2000).

In this article we focus on overcoming this barrier of distrust of the medical system, which can influence the participation of older African Americans into clinical research. We draw from our own study investigating the relationship between psychosocial factors and increases in hypertension risk factors in older African Americans. We outline four types of trust that we found to be essential to successful recruitment. We also present the relative effectiveness of various methods used to recruit older African Americans. These methods fall into three broad categories that include phone and mailing strategies, direct community outreach, and use of the media.

BRIEF OVERVIEW OF THE STUDY

This study was one of four in the National Institute on Aging (NIA)-funded Duke Center for Exploratory Studies in Older Minorities. Participants were 148 African Americans with normal blood pressure, and 18 with hypertension, aged 40 to 65 years of age. Participants were required to be studied in a hospital psychophysiologic laboratory environment; eat prepared meals in a hospital clinical research unit; collect 24-hour physiologic measures; complete a battery of questionnaires; participate in interviews and focus groups; and participate in other data collection procedures to construct new, culturally sensitive measures of stress, perceived racism, and social support.

Recruiting Volunteers: Selected Factors Affecting Likelihood of Participation

The recruitment of volunteers to participate in research is nearly always a challenging endeavor. As illustrated in this volume, it can be especially challenging to recruit many ethnic minority populations, given the history of distrust of biomedical research. At the same time, however, ethnic minorities, especially African Americans, are likely being recruited and are participating in research in historic numbers, owing in part to NIH-mandated inclusion guidelines. Successful recruitment of African American participants does not happen automatically, and researchers should be aware of potential factors that might increase or decrease the likelihood of finding volunteers. In our experience, at least three factors seem to be critical for successful recruitment: (1) The degree of physiological or psychological invasiveness of the research procedures (e.g., from surveys to surgical procedures); (2) the convenience (or inconvenience) to the volunteer of participating; and (3) the trust that has been established between the researcher/research institution and the community at large.

In fact, it might be possible to predict the likelihood of potential volunteers agreeing to participate in a study by examining the interaction of the three aforementioned dimensions. Table 1 shows the three dimensions of participation. Any given study can be rated as "low," "moderate," or "high" along each dimension. For example, a study could be low in invasiveness (e.g., a survey of general knowledge), high in convenience (a phone survey), and from an institution or researchers high in trust (e.g., a long-standing and respectful relationship with the community). Each of these dimensions and ratings can be scored based on their likelihood of increasing participation, where a "3": means "highly likely"; a "2" means "moderately likely"; and a "1" means "least likely." The ways in which these dimensions interact to predict participation are illustrated in Table 2.

BUILDING TRUST

Going into this research we were very conscious of the possibility that African Americans in our community might view the majority population, as well as traditionally White institutions, with suspicion and mistrust. In addition, we were aware that cultural differences between African Americans and White Americans might make trusting difficult. We also knew from experience, however, that even in cases where the ethnicity of the recruiter or experimenter is the same as that of the participant, other factors such as differences in socioeconomic status and simply being an "unknown entity" to the participant community may present challenges to building trust.

Therefore, it was our belief that the most important initial strategy for successful recruitment was to build trust with the participant community. More specifically, our goals were to establish trust between the participants/community leaders/community gatekeepers and the investigators/recruiters/and Duke as an institution. We were also working with the community to build trust in the study project, the scientific process, and that the data and results would be interpreted correctly and reported in an accurate and ethical manner. Finally, we wanted to build trust that the benefits of collaborating with us on research would endure in the community beyond the length of the study. The following strategies were used to build trust in each of these areas.

Building Trust in Recruiters, Experimenters, and the Institution

We believed that one of the most powerful tools in building trust was to select a recruitment team and lead recruiters who already had or could readily foster a positive rapport with the participant community. Creating a recruitment team that comprised African American individuals who were similar to the participant sample in age, gender, and socioeconomic status, lived in the community, and who were known, trusted, and respected also was essential. That these recruiters were trusted and respected by the African American community greatly facilitated access to community members.

Building Trust in Community Leaders and Gatekeepers, and Engaging Them in Recruitment

Similarly, we found it important to build trust with community leaders. We needed these individuals to help establish our credibility with the community and to recruit participants. These individuals operated as community gatekeepers in that they influenced access to participants. They also had the expertise to educate both the African American and White (experimenter and institution) communities about cultural similarities and differences between the groups. They were central to building trusting and respectful relationships between groups—both the African American and experimenter/institution groups, as well as subgroups within the African American community. Of importance was the fact that our recruitment and investigative teams had established a history of trust in the community based on several years of reputable and beneficial community research and service prior to the start of this study. This created an advantageous carry-over effect.

Building Trust in the Study

It has been our experience that among the minority lay community research is often viewed with suspicion, as not relevant to the community, and as sometimes misrepresentative or exploitative. Therefore, we felt that in order to succeed it was essential to create trust in the value and credibility of the study. To accomplish this, we presented our study as part of the larger study of the Duke Center for Exploratory Studies in Older Minorities. We emphasized that the Center had been created expressly to serve and promote health in the area's minority communities. We also stressed that the Center's projects were directed and conducted by minority investigators who understood the culture and issues of the community, and that the Center itself consisted not only of Duke but of a consortium of institutions including area Black churches and North Carolina Central University, an historically Black university. Emphasizing these aspects of the Center's structure and function helped build community trust in the study and in the individuals/institutions involved with it.

Building Trust in the Scientific Process

Minority communities often express concern that health studies with minority groups are devised by scientists who lack a true understanding of the minority community (Brink, 1994). As a result, minority communities often believe that such studies perpetuate misperceptions of the community, and that these misperceptions end up taking on a scientific legitimacy (Flores, Castro, & Fernandez-Esquer, 1995). To address these concerns, we considered it important that gatekeepers and participants have trust in the scientific process itself. To do so, we involved participants in the scientific process by soliciting their feedback regarding methods (particularly qualitative methods), procedures, and the construction of culturally sensitive scales to measure social support, stress, and perceived racism. Input was obtained through both informal and formal methods. Informal methods included soliciting feedback at each step of the study (e.g., sample collection, eating prepared meals, etc.) and changes were made as deemed appropriate. Formal procedures included interviews, focus groups, and semi-structured questionnaires. Participant input guided our thinking, the development of instruments, the interpretation of the data, and considerations of future directions. At the same time, participants and the community indicated to us that they felt they were a valued part of the process and had a concrete impact on the study. The net result of this high degree of participant feedback, we believe, was enhanced faith in the particular procedures being used.

Building Trust That Data and Results Be Interpreted and Reported Accurately and Ethically

As suggested earlier, a common complaint of minorities is that the data collected from them are often misinterpreted, misrepresent the community, or worst of all, can be used against the community. Indeed, a number of our participants expressed these concerns and inquired as to who would be interpreting the data and exactly how they were to be used. Several people also asked about the ethnicity of the investigators. To address these concerns and the potential barriers to recruitment and retention that they created, the research team took particular care to acknowledge that the participants' concerns were valid, and to fully and carefully answer all questions. It was particularly important to reiterate that our purpose was to serve and help promote the health of the community, and that data would be interpreted as accurately as possible. We also emphasized that the information we had obtained from participants through qualitative methods would be very important to data interpretation, and that the former would have access to the results as they became available.

Building Trust That Long-Term Effects Would Continue Beyond the Duration of the Study

We realize that the community was concerned that investigators not simply take from the community but also leave behind something that the community "owned." Although we could not guarantee that initiatives of the grant would continue beyond the duration of the grant, our Center attempted to develop and establish programs that would extend autonomously beyond the duration of the grant. This was part of building the community infrastructure for research, discussed earlier. Examples of this include the NCCU and church-based project where church members were rewarded for engaging in health-promoting behaviors. Another spin-off project from the Center grant was an "Afrobics Exercise" project (combining traditional African dance with aerobic exercise) that has been conducted in community centers and churches and continues now without federal support (i.e., participants pay out-of-pocket for classes). One of these churches also requested that we add classes in T'ai Chi and Meditation for Health, activities that are now under way with the help of one of the investigators. Another example is the Lincoln Community Health Center Stress Management Program that provided free stress-management group sessions for persons served by the community center—additional support that our commitment to the health of its members was not temporary.

The steps outlined above, we believe, resulted in a high rate of recruitment and retention success—building trust in the recruitment team, experimenters, institution, the study, and with gatekeepers, helped optimize the effectiveness of the specific recruitment strategies described below.

OVERVIEW OF RECRUITMENT STRATEGIES

A variety of recruitment strategies was employed, focusing on calls and mailings, face-to-face community outreach, and use of the media. These strategies included making "cold calls" using the U.S. Census data, accessing the DUMC Center for Aging Subject Registry, contacting senior centers and residential facilities, approaching physicians, conducting blood pressure screenings, and hosting visits to the laboratory and DUMC. We also contacted government and community organizations, African American fraternities and sororities, Black-owned businesses, African American community organizations, and African American churches to engage their support and assistance with recruitment efforts. Using public media (television and radio talk shows, newspapers, newsletters, flyers, etc.) also was an effective means of recruiting. During the second year of the grant we discovered that changing the exclusionary and age criteria, as well as participant reimbursement, significantly enhanced recruitment. We will now describe each of these strategies in detail, as well as their relative success in recruiting participants.

Telephone and Mail Recruitment Strategies

Census. One of our initial approaches to recruitment from May through November of the first year of the grant was to make "cold calls" to individuals sampled from the 1990 Census. Our research team received training in phone solicitation from Johnston and Zabor, a company in Research Triangle Park, NC. Although a total of 645 outgoing calls were made during the first-year period from May through November, the response rate was low.

No participants were recruited from these efforts. Despite our best efforts, we realized that regardless of the community, "cold calls" were one of the least likely strategies of fostering trust and engaging participation.

Center for the Study of Aging and Human Development Subject Registry. During the first months of the grant, we also turned to the Duke Center for Aging registry of individuals. This registry comprised several thousand individuals who had volunteered to have their names placed in the registry, indicating they were interested in being contacted for future studies. Approximately 1,000 African Americans were listed in the registry at the time of the study, but based on the registry data only a handful seemed to fit the inclusion criteria. These individuals were contacted, but none ultimately qualified due to health conditions that excluded them from the study.

Direct, Face-To-Face Community Outreach Strategies

Noting the poor results from the phone contacts, we changed our strategies in July to employ more direct, face-to-face recruitment in the community. The idea was that face-to-face contact would allow more opportunities to build trust through personal, eye-to-eye contact, open dialogue, and addressing individual concerns and questions. These strategies included establishing a network of community recruitment contacts; putting together a slide presentation on the Center for use in speaking engagements; approaching senior citizen centers; using public media (television, radio, newspapers, newsletters, flyers, etc.); engaging leaders and gatekeepers in the Black community to assist with recruitment; approaching Black-owned businesses; recruiting at African American community organizations; soliciting fraternities and sororities; visiting and recruiting from African American churches; and approaching physicians about referrals. We continued conducting the phone recruitment from the Census list but in a reduced fashion compared to previous months. From August through December of the first year of the grant, we registered an additional 114 contacts from these outreach efforts and recruited and studied 15 participants.

These direct, face-to-face recruitment efforts were far more effective than the "cold call" and mailing strategies. Clearly, making the effort to meet and talk with potential participants, answer questions, allay fears and concerns, and have visual and physical contact, strongly facilitated trust and participation in the study. Although it may appear that the face-to-face trust-building may be extremely time consuming and labor intensive, which indeed it is, it was clear that the cost-benefit ratio of these strategies was far better those that provided by the "cold calls."

Senior Citizen Centers. Encouraged by the initial response to the face-to-face recruitment, we began our second year with outreach efforts directed toward senior citizen centers. We soon discovered that although the interest was high, the health criteria of our study (normal, healthy, medication-free African Americans 60 years and older) prevented many individuals from participating. (This issue is discussed in greater detail below.) Nonetheless, we approached five predominantly African American senior citizen residences; presented a brief talk about cardiovascular disease and hypertension in African Americans; described the Center and our study; and addressed questions and concerns. Although 11 individuals indicated interest in participating, none qualified due to medical reasons.

Physicians as Referral Sources. Our team also mailed letters and made calls and office visits to physicians (especially African American physicians) in the hope that they would refer potential participants to our study. Several physicians were receptive to this idea and referred some patients. Most, however, stated that they either did not have the staffing power to make those referrals and were concerned about putting their patients at risk because of their poor health status, or that they were not willing to refer their patients to research studies in general. One physician openly expressed his suspicion of research as the basis of his reluctance to refer.

Blood Pressure Screenings and Health Fairs. Our research team regularly performed blood pressure screenings in the community and manned booths at health fairs to recruit participants. These efforts provided face-to-face opportunities for dialogue and relationship building, and each event typically resulted in about 15-25 interested individuals. Despite this interest, however, the exclusionary health criteria prevented many of these individuals from joining the study.

Hosting Visits to DUMC, the Laboratory, and the Rankin Clinical Research Unit. Several church and community groups indicated that they were interested in visiting our facilities and learning more about the research taking place at DUMC—evidence of our success at building community relationships as well as generating interest and support of the mission and the work of the Center. After arranging for several visits from various community groups, 10 individuals were interested in participating, but once again health conditions excluded them from participation.

African American Churches. Approximately 20 traditionally Black churches were contacted for recruitment purposes. The research team phoned the churches and asked whether information about the study could be placed in the church bulletin or announced at the Sunday sermon. Several recruiters visited or attended church services. All churches contacted were receptive and most followed up with posting or announcing our information. Several churches invited members of our team to deliver talks on health topics to some of the senior church groups, and at the same time inform them of the projects at the Center. We were delighted to respond to these requests, and believe that our work with area churches not only furthered our trust-building efforts, but enhanced the credibility of our commitment to give back to the community. Few actual participants, however, were recruited using this method, again due to poor health status.

Changing Participant Criteria and Reimbursement. It became apparent from our intensive recruitment efforts and low enrollment rate (15 participants qualified out of nearly 700 contacts) that despite the successful trust building and resultant interest generated in participating, the poor health status of the participants was a primary factor preventing their participation in the study. This should have been no surprise to us in view of the well-documented findings indicating that, relative to Whites, African Americans suffer disproportionately higher rates of all major diseases and more severe consequences of such, and that the aging process may be accelerated in African Americans. Thus, we decided to make judicious changes in the age, health, and medication criteria of the study, and to increase the monetary reimbursement to participants. The original criteria held that participants were to be African Americans 60 years of age or older, with no history of illness and being medication free. These are relatively stringent inclusion criteria. We lowered the age range first to 50 and older, and still encountered difficulties finding participants who met the health criteria. After several more months of difficulty, we dropped the age criteria to include individuals 40 and older. In addition, we changed the health criteria to include those who were free of illness at the time of the study and had no history of serious illnesses. We also changed the medication criteria to include those on antihypertensive medications. Lastly, we increased the subject reimbursement from $100 to $200. All of these changes significantly increased our recruitment success rate for subsequent years of the grant.

Thus, an important lesson we learned was that given the significantly higher illness rates among older African Americans, healthy, older African American participants were extraordinarily difficult to identify and recruit. This issue is particularly important in psychophysiologic research where health status and medical conditions importantly affect outcomes. Hence, in conducting such research, careful consideration of the reality-based impact of age, health, and medication criteria on recruitment procedures, timelines, and budget is essential.

Government and Community Organizations. After changing our age, health, and medication criteria, a number of government and community organizations were contacted for assistance with recruitment. All were responsive to our inquiries and provided opportunities for us to dialogue and build trust through talks, blood pressure screenings, and speaking with potential participants at their sites. Examples of the organizations approached include the Durham Committee on the Affairs of Black People, Durham County Social Services, Durham County Health Department, Lincoln Community Health Center, and the Durham Housing Authority. These efforts would successfully yield three to five potential participants per effort.

Sororities and Fraternal Organizations. Seven sororities and fraternities were also approached for recruitment of participants. The research team gave talks at organizational meetings, informed individuals about the Center and its studies, and invited their participation. Although individuals indicated much interest and excitement in the study, only three were able to commit to participation. We suspect the reason for this low rate may have been that members of these organizations were very socially and politically active and may have found it difficult to commit to a study involving such significant amounts of time and energy.

Word-of-Mouth Recruitment. Many participants were recruited by word-of-mouth from other participants who had completed this or other studies at the Center. This strategy was one of our strongest and most successful efforts. We believe its strength was due to the strong trust and rapport we had established with our participants, and the benefits they reported having experienced from participation which in turn motivated them to invite others into the effort.

Black-Owned Businesses. A variety of Black-owned businesses were contacted for recruitment purposes. Members of the research team would set up a time to meet with the owner or employer, discuss the mission and purpose of the Center, and describe the study and benefits for participants. We would then often do a blood pressure screening or presentation to employees, speak with potential participants, and leave literature describing the study (e.g., fliers, etc.). Responses from Black-owned business proprietors were positive and supportive, with some owners actually offering to sponsor our study or financially contribute to our program. That these community leaders were willing to "put their money" behind our initiative showed strong support and trust in what was being accomplished together in partnership. Approximately 135 contacts with interested individuals were made through our business outreach recruitment efforts.

Posting Fliers and Notices. Another successful recruitment strategy was that of posting fliers and notices. The research team posted fliers throughout the Duke hospitals and clinics and at the Veteran's Administration Hospital. Notices were also placed on employee pay stubs. Fliers were posted throughout the community at shopping centers, businesses, bus stations, the public library, restaurants, community bulletin boards, etc. Other than our face-to-face contacts with the community and use of the media, this recruitment strategy was by far the most successful in producing participants. We believe the reason this strategy was successful was in part due to participant self-selection (individuals were motivated by their own initiative to contact us), and in part because they had an opportunity to talk with us, ask questions, allay fears, and in essence, build trust. Approximately 50% of our sample were recruited in this manner.

Media Strategies

Television, Radio, and Newspapers. The media was also quite helpful in informing the public of our study and recruiting participants. Six radio stations broadcast public service announcements and hosted radio call-in talk shows in which we were involved. During the talk shows, investigators provided information about the significance of hypertension and cardiovascular disease in African Americans; discussed the purpose of the Duke NIA-funded Center; emphasized that the Duke Center was a consortium of institutions including a local historically Black University (North Carolina Central University) and area Black churches; and described the specific study intent and procedures, along with the benefits of participating. Listeners were invited to call in with general questions about stress and heart disease, and were given information as to how to enroll in the study.

In addition, we worked with two local television stations to recruit participants through the medical report sections of their news broadcasts, and advertised our studies using the free cable television broadcasting. We also placed ads in general and Black local newspapers; listed our study in the community bulletin board sections of papers; and wrote articles for the papers describing our initiatives. Information about the study was also published in citizens' and business newsletters, or inserts with utility bills.

Because these strategies involved the sharing of information and opportunities for contact, dialogue, and relationship building, interest and involvement in the study was greatly facilitated. These strategies, successfully yielded an average of 5-10 calls per effort.

SUMMARY

Our team made nearly a thousand "contacts" with participants, each of which involved one or more of the following: an introductory phone call, bringing the participant into the lab, taking a medical history, and administering a physical examination. Hundreds more contacts were made where the participant was excluded on the initial contact, most often due to health reasons. Of these contacts, 148 participants completed the study: 120 women and 28 men, 130 normotensives and 18 hypertensives.

Overall, our most successful recruitment strategies were those that involved opportunities to build trust. We described several areas in which we felt it was important to foster trust: among recruiters, experimenters, institutions; with community leaders and gatekeepers; in the study project and scientific process; in the data-reporting process. To foster trust that the benefits of collaboration would endure in the community beyond the length of the study was of utmost importance.

Trust building and optimal recruitment response was best achieved by strategies involving face-to-face contact with potential participants. These strategies included establishing a network of community recruitment contacts; making presentations; approaching senior citizen centers; approaching Black physicians for referrals;

conducting blood pressure screenings and recruiting at health fairs; arranging visits to Duke and the Center; recruiting at African American churches; approaching leaders and gatekeepers in the Black community, organizations, and government to assist with recruitment; using public media (television, radio, newspapers, newsletters, flyers, etc.); soliciting fraternities and sororities; relying on word-of-mouth from previous participants; and soliciting the support of Black-owned businesses.

With respect to effectiveness, least successful were the "cold calls" from the Census listing, Aging Center subject registry, and physician referrals. We believe these strategies involved a minimal amount of trust and relationship building, and hence yielded a minimal response rate. Most successful were the strategies allowing for the greatest direct contact and dialogue, which seemed to increase the likelihood for trusting, respectful relationships. These strategies consisted of engaging the support of Black-owned businesses; approaching leaders and gatekeepers in the Black community and government to assist with recruitment; support of the media (television and radio talk shows, newspapers, fliers, etc.); and word-of-mouth from participants in the study.

We also wish to point to the importance of health status and age in conducting research with older African Americans, keeping in mind that illness rates are significantly higher among older African Americans compared to Whites, and that healthy older African American participants may be extremely difficult to locate. Hence, careful consideration of age, health, and medication criteria is essential in designing and conducting such research, and accounting for these issues in recruitment procedures, timelines, and budget is critical to the success of the study.

Lastly, readers may also note that despite the fact that our research team had a long history of successful recruitment and strong rapport in the minority community, it nonetheless took approximately 1 year to identify appropriate recruitment resources for this particular project, and to build the infrastructure of trusting relationships within this network of resources. A lesson we learned is that a critical aspect of recruitment success is realistic planning and budgeting of time, staffing, and money required for this necessary preliminary work. We hope our discussion of some of the challenges and the presentation of strategies used to overcome these challenges will be helpful to investigators attempting to conduct research with minority populations.

REFERENCES

American Cancer Society. (1989). *Cancer and the poor: A report to the nation and findings of regional hearings.* Atlanta, GA: Author.

Brawley, O. W., & Tejeda, H. (1995). Minority inclusion in clinical trials: Issues and potential strategies. *Journal of National Cancer Institute Monographs, 17,* 55-57.

Brink, T. L. (1994). The need for qualitative research on mental health of elder Hispanics. *International Journal of Aging and Human Development, 38,* 279-291.

el-Sadr, W., & Capps, L. (1992). The challenge of minority recruitment in clinical trials for AIDS. *Journal of the American Medical Association, 267,* 954-957.

Flores, E. T., Castro, F. G., & Fernandez-Esquer, M. E. (1995). Social theory, social action, and intervention research: Implications for cancer prevention among Latinos. *Journal of the National Cancer Institute Monographs, 18,* 101-108.

Lenfant, C. (1995). Enhancing minority participation in research: The NHLBI experience. *Circulation, 92,* 279-280.

Levkoff, S. E., Levy, B., & Weitzman, P. F. (in press). The role of ethnicity and religion in the help seeking of family caregivers. *Journal of Cross-Cultural Gerontology.*

Levkoff, S. E., Levy, B., & Weitzman, P. F. (2000). The matching model of recruitment. *Journal of Mental Health and Aging, 6*(1), 29-38.

National Institutes of Health guidelines on inclusion of women and minorities as subjects in clinical research, Part VIII. Fed. Reg (1994, March 28).

Thomas, S. B., & Quinn, S. C. (1991). The Tuskegee Syphilis Study 1932 to 1972: Implications for HIV education and AIDS risk education programs in the black community. *American Journal of Public Health, 81,* 1498-1504.

Acknowledgments. This research was conducted under the auspices of the Exploratory Center for Minority Aging and Health Promotion and supported by the National Institute on Aging (Grant # P20 AG12058) and the Office for Research on Minority Health of the National Institutes of Health. Norman B. Anderson's contribution does not represent the opinions of the National Institutes of Health, the Department of Health and Human Services, or the Federal Government.

Offprints. Requests for offprints should be directed to Maya McNeilly, PhD, Duke University Medical Center, Durham, NC 27710.

Journal of Mental Health and Aging, Vol. 6, No. 1, 2000

The Power of Labels: Recruiting Dementia-Affected Chinese American Elders and Their Caregivers

Zibin Guo, PhD
University of Tennessee, Chattanooga, TN

Becca R. Levy, PhD
Yale University School of Medicine New Haven, CT

W. Ladson Hinton, MD
University of California, Davis Medical Center

Patricia Flynn Weitzman, PhD
Sue E. Levkoff, ScD
Harvard Medical School, Boston, MA

Recruiting Chinese American participants into studies of Alzheimer's disease and dementia can be particularly challenging because of the powerful social stigma attached to mental illness in Chinese cultures. In this article, we describe experiences recruiting Chinese American individuals into a cross-cultural qualitative study of dementia caregiving. Based on multiple sources of data from caregivers who participated in our study, those who declined participation, and Chinese American health care providers, we have identified a process of dementia-label avoidance engaged in by both Chinese American families and health care providers. We describe how this process can interfere with the recruitment of Chinese American participants into studies of mental illness and offer strategies for enhancing recruitment success.

Recruiting dementia-affected minority elders and their family caregivers to participate in research can be challenging. A wide range of barriers to minority participation in health research has been documented (e.g., Caban, 1995; Young, Edevie, Young, & Peters, 1996). In our own research on culture and caregiving, a significant obstacle to minority recruitment has proven to be a mismatch between the assumptions and goals held by researchers, and those held by members of ethnic minorities (Levkoff, Levy, & Weitzman, 2000). A precursor to a good collaborative match between the goals of health researchers and the goals of minority participants is a better understanding by researchers of the cultural factors that can influence the health of minority individuals. Factors unique to Chinese cultural responses to dementing illness have started to be identified (e.g., Elliott, Di Minno, Lam, & Tu, 1996; Hinton & Levkoff, in press), but few studies examine the ways in which the label of dementia is responded to by Chinese Americans, and how the social significance of the label of dementia may impact the willingness of Chinese American families and health care providers to participate in studies of Alzheimer's disease and related disorders (ADRD). This article attempts to fill that gap by describing the ways in which dementia was viewed by Chinese American caregivers and health care providers who participated in a cross-cultural study of caregiving.

Our analysis of the data from our cross-cultural studies led us to identify a social process of dementia-label avoidance among Chinese Americans. This process occurs because of a cultural tendency for Chinese communities to stigmatize both the individual and their family if a mental illness, such as dementia, becomes publicly known (Elliott et al., 1996; Li & Lin, 1981). Thus, when a family suspects that an elder has dementia, the following process may take place: (1) the family actively avoids the dementia label being suggested for the elder by providers and instead tries to normalize dementia as part of the aging process; (2) some Chinese health care providers may cooperate with families in their avoidance of a formal diagnosis of dementia to protect the family from stigmatization. Because of this process, dementia researchers are likely to encounter difficulty in recruiting Chinese American families. The following discussion will briefly outline the social meaning attached to mental illness in Chinese culture, and will detail research findings which led us to identify this process of dementia-label avoidance. We argue that dementia researchers need to be aware of the power of mental illness labels in Chinese communities to develop effective recruitment strategies, and conclude with recommendations on how researchers can develop such strategies.

Mental Illness in Chinese Cultures

A major contribution of the field of anthropology to health promotion is identification of the ways in which cultural and social contexts can shape illness experiences. It has been documented that various cultures classify illness according to different criteria (Fabrega, 1991; Kleinman, 1980). Stigma, which is the act of conferring on a person a set of powerful negative images, can be one of the cultural constructions associated with certain behaviors, including illness behaviors (Fabrega, 1991). Different illness labels often evoke different levels of stigma within a given culture (Bhugra, 1989; Mansouri & Dowell, 1989; Rabin, Rosser, & Butler, 1993). A criticism of the western system of psychiatric illness categorization is that it fails to recognize social and cultural factors, such as stigmatization, which can influence the nature of symptomatology and how illness is experienced by an individual and his/her family (Rush, 1996).

Compared with the more dichotomous way in which western medicine tends to separate illness from its emotional and social context, traditional Chinese medicine describes mind and body as an integrated whole (Li, 1986; Unschuld, 1981), with mental imbalance giving rise to physical illness (Li & Lin, 1981). Although Chinese medicine focuses its pathology, diagnosis, disease classification and treatment predominantly on physiological problems, the quality of one's mental condition is central to one's physiological condition. An 'excess of emotions' is held as one initial cause of physiological disorders (Li & Lin, 1981). Major Chinese philosophical traditions such as Taoism and Confucianism reinforce this view of illness by emphasizing the ability to regulate emotions as a prerequisite to psychological harmony with nature and human society (Li & Lin, 1981; Tseng, 1995). Supernatural explanations, such as spirit possession and sorcery, are also incorporated into Chinese cultural beliefs about psychiatric disorders (Lin, 1981).

Symptoms which can be defined as dementia related by western standards are found in two contrasting classifications of cognitive problems in the Chinese medical literature. Though the criteria for defining and categorizing these symptoms often overlap, they have distinct meanings. The two categories are: Jian-wan Zheng (forgetfulness syndrome) and Zhi Dai Zheng (senile mental retardation—dementia). Jian-wan Zheng mainly implies symptoms related to the decline of memory caused by aging (Wang, 1989), while Zhi Dai Zheng denotes symptoms related to mental illness caused by a failure to regulate one's emotions or by excessive drinking and smoking (Li, 1986). Zhi Dai Zheng is more serious and stigmatizing, comparable to such major psychiatric disorders as schizophrenia (Li, 1986). The stigma of mental illness and the ambiguousness of dementia-related definitions in Chinese medicine taken together seem to result in a Chinese cultural tendency to normalize memory loss, and minimize the significance of "uncharacteristic" behaviors in the elderly (Elliott et al., 1996). In her field study conducted in China, Ikels (1998) observed:

> . . . a test score indicative of mild dementia that would trigger alarm bells and possibly panic in most Americans would mean little or nothing to an elderly Chinese because the latter would not perceive the symptoms that generated the score as particularly disabling. Alternatively he or she might recognize them as disabling, but not as abnormal for an older person and, therefore, as not worth getting excited about (p. 260).

Although the practice of modern psychiatry appeared in Chinese society as early as the 1930s, mostly it consisted of fragmented individual practices (Kleinman, 1986). The formal practice of clinical psychiatry and the systematic study of dementia are still relatively new to Chinese society. For example, it was only as recent as 1984 that the first Chinese Classification of Mental Disease (CCMD) was established by a fledgling community of Chinese practitioners of western psychiatry. The existence of this community may slowly alter the ways in which dementia is viewed in Chinese society. Thus far, however, its impact on the cultural beliefs of the Chinese mainland population appears minimal. With this cultural background information in mind, we will now describe our cross-cultural study, and discuss how Chinese culturally derived labels of dementia gave rise to recruitment challenges.

STUDY

Sample and Methods

Our data came from retrospective qualitative interviews (including field notes) with 16 Chinese-American caregivers who were successfully recruited into our cross-cultural study of dementia caregiving conducted through the NIA-funded Exploratory Center for Research on Health Promotion in Older Minority Populations at Harvard Medical School. We also analyzed field notes based on another 14 Chinese-American caregivers who participated in a quantitative study of caregiving, and semistructured interviews with 3 Chinese-American physicians and 2 community-based Chinese American nurses. In addition, we analyzed detailed field notes taken during the recruitment phase of our qualitative study, including notes taken during several recruitment interviews with individuals who refused participation. Our criteria for recruitment of caregivers for the retrospective qualitative interviews were: (1) that the caregiver be an adult family member who self-identified as providing substantial day-to-day care of a family member with diagnosed or probable ADRD within the past year (caregivers of elders placed in nursing homes during the preceding year were eligible); (2) that the caregiver be Chinese or Chinese-American.

Most of the Chinese-American families successfully recruited for the qualitative and quantitative study live in Boston's Chinatown. Elders and caregivers were ethnically Chinese immigrants from mainland China, Vietnam, Burma, Hong Kong, and Taiwan, most of whom came to the United States in the 1980s. While there was considerable diversity in education and occupational status in this sample, a significant minority of the caregivers and their elders had little formal education, with the caregivers typically working here as unskilled laborers. Most elders had medical coverage, including Medicaid and Medicare. A few of the families came from suburban towns around Boston. Caregivers in this group were more highly educated, and included physicians, accountants, engineers, and academics. Most of their elderly parents were relatively recent immigrants (usually here 10 years or less), and had come to the U.S. under their children's sponsorship, often to care for grandchildren.

The 16 qualitative interviews were conducted by two interviewers, with one taking the lead and the other taking field notes. In all cases, there was a linguistic match between the lead interviewer and the caregiver; however, no systematic effort was made to match interviewers on the basis of ethnicity, race or gender. All interviews were conducted in the caregiver's native language and the setting of their choice, which was usually the caregiver's home. Interviewers used a guide that outlined domains of interest, including current social context, description of illness onset and course, interpretations of illness and symptoms, day-to-day caregiving activities, experiences and activities associated with caregiving, and ideals of aging. Social context included family members living with the caregiver and with the elder; family members involved in caregiving and/or decision making about the elder; family and nonfamily sources of social support; and contact with service providers. Interviewers were not given specific questions to ask, and had considerable latitude to explore other domains that emerged during the interview. Sessions lasted from 1 to 5 hours. Interviews were completed in 1 or 2 visits, depending upon the preference of the caregiver. All were taped, transcribed and, if necessary, translated into English. Detailed field notes for each interview provided descriptions of the setting and nonverbal aspects of the interview process.

Data Analysis

Qualitative interview transcripts and field notes were content analyzed, a process which consists primarily of coding and summarizing the occurrence of specific forms of content (Grinnell, 1994). We coded transcripts and field notes for idioms and illness labels used by caregivers to describe dementia-related symptoms. Interview transcripts were also analyzed for evaluative clauses, that is, statements about the nature or cause of the dementia-related symptoms. Evaluative clauses can give direct insights into the primary labels that shape the way people think and behave in their daily lives, and the meanings attached to those labels (Luborsky, 1994). We examined evaluative clauses to uncover the meaning attached to mental illness and dementia labels used by caregivers. In our interviews with health care providers, we content-analyzed parts of the interview that revealed information about their attitudes and practices related to diagnosing ADRD in their Chinese patients, and their attitudes toward referring patients for study participation. We also content-analyzed notes taken during recruitment interviews with individuals who refused participation.

RESULTS

Numerous themes emerged in the qualitative interviews, as well as numerous content categories from both field notes and interviews. For the purposes of this article, we focus exclusively on those themes and content areas having to do with recruitment obstacles and associated participant perceptions. Discussions of other themes and topics from these data can be found elsewhere (Hicks & Lam, in press; Hinton & Levkoff, in press; Levkoff, Levy, & Weitzman, in press; Weitzman, Chee, & Levkoff, 1999). Here we will present themes and content areas together, along with supporting examples and quotations.

Labels as a Barrier to Caregiver Recruitment

Over the 4-year period of the qualitative and quantitative studies, we conducted various recruitment initiatives in Boston's urban and suburban Chinese American communities. These efforts included contacting home care agencies, churches, and several Chinese Sunday schools to refer families with an ADRD elder. We also offered free memory screenings through a local newsletter and radio talk show. Over 200 Chinese American individuals came to be tested. Through analysis of notes taken during recruitment interviews and field notes documenting the behavior of individuals who came for the memory screenings, a topic emerged having to do with a strong resistance to acknowledging the presence of dementia. For example, during the memory screenings our researchers noted that most individuals came in two stages. Individuals would first come to ask questions about the screening, but decline to be screened. Later that day or another day, most of these individuals came back for screening. This widespread hesitance about coming for a memory screening seemed to be explained by a woman who had severe memory problems and required family assistance to accomplish everyday activities of living, but was unwilling to participate in the study because she said: "If other people know about this, my grandchildren will have difficulties to get married." Similarly a caregiver who inquired about our screening activities explained why she would not participate in the study:

> . . . well, he does have some problems. But I do not think they are serious problem, at least they are not as big as he is trying to think of . . . every old people has some difficulties with their memory. When they are getting old, of course their Ji Yi Li (memory function) will not be as good as they were younger. That is nature. But the worst thing is to make him worry about it even more. . . . Can you tell me is there a solution to this? I do not think so. It is not a new phenomena, and people have been living with it for long time. It is just like being old. No one likes being old,

> especially in here (United States). But is being old a problem, is there a solution? If there is not, why we should believe it is a problem. I do not want him to think he has a problem . . .

We found a similar level of refusal from families recruited through home care agencies. Many of these families expressed great alarm when we contacted them, sometimes denying that they had an ADRD elder and asking not to be contacted again. Even though we explained that participation in the study could be beneficial and that information would be kept confidential, most caregivers refused. As one caregiver put it: "It is family thing, [we] do not want to talk about it to outsider, please understand." The hesitant, two-stage approach to our memory screening by so many, as well as the widely unsuccessful recruitment interviews, seemed to reflect heightened fear of ADRD due, in part, to the strong stigma associated with mental disorders in Chinese cultures. With caregivers from each of the other three study groups recruited in a similar fashion (African American, Latino, and Irish American), we encountered significantly less recruitment refusal.

Labels as Barriers to Health Care Provider Participation

At the outset of the study, we worked closely with Chinese American primary care physicians who worked with Chinese elders in and around Boston. Despite their expressed willingness to support the study, we found that several months into our recruitment efforts, few had actually referred any patients. Among the 16 elders who ultimately enrolled in the study all screened with cognitive impairments highly suggestive of ADRD, yet none had a formal diagnosis from their physicians. Of these 16 individuals, only two were referred by their Chinese American physicians. Caregivers who participated in the qualitative interview commonly reported that their Chinese American physicians told them that the memory loss or confusion in the caregiver's elder was just a normal part of aging.

When we recognized that our efforts to recruit participants through their Chinese American providers had been largely unsuccessful, we went back to providers to ask questions that might help us understand why our efforts had failed. We conducted semistructured interviews with 3 Chinese American primary care physicians and 2 Chinese American nurses. Thematic analyses of the interviews revealed a theme of discounting the value of ADRD study participation. Four beliefs seemed to lead providers to discount the value of ADRD study participation for their Chinese-American patients. These beliefs were: (1) the western diagnostic criteria are vague and cannot be easily interpreted, so it is hard for providers to identify individuals with ADRD; (2) if violent behavior is not present in the elder, there is no need to make a diagnosis and initiate treatment; (3) Chinese American families usually can provide adequate support for ADRD elders and do not require outside assistance; (4) study participation and/or diagnosis provide no significant benefits to most families and elders, and could add to their strain by inflicting social stigma.

Label Awareness in Families Who Did Participate

As already stated, none of the 16 families who ultimately participated in the qualitative study had a formal diagnosis for their elder. Although our recruitment interviews informed us that most caregivers were aware of the biomedical terms for the disease, for example, Alzheimer's or dementia, few would use those terms during the interviews. A theme emerged in the qualitative interviews of attributing the elder's symptoms to advanced age, rather than ADRD (see Hinton & Levkoff, in press). For example, Dr. B., a Chinese American physician and caregiver had taken her elderly mother to neurologists and psychiatrists who, in all likelihood, told Dr. B. her mother had ADRD. Despite her own biomedical understanding of disease processes, Dr. B. never used the words Alzheimer's or dementia, and framed her mother's illness as a normal part of the aging process, stating: "I see it as a part of what happens, I guess, as one gets older. That is how I see it, it's just what happens." Another caregiver stated explicitly that she would rather to use her own terms for ADRD because the biomedical ones "were too sensitive."

Aside from advanced age, another theme around symptom attribution emerged in the data. This theme had to do with explaining the elders' symptoms as being caused by hardships experienced earlier in life, such as deaths of loved ones, family conflicts, trauma caused by the political upheaval of China's Cultural Revolution, and stressful living conditions. One caregiver explained that her husband had suffered a great deal during China's Cultural Revolution, causing him to be "thinking, thinking, and thinking about the events in the past, and as a result he became all bad . . . he thought about things until he went all crazy . . . his brain is hurt and his psyche is wounded . . ." (See Hinton & Levkoff, in press, for further explication of nonmedical attributions for disease processes found in this data set.) Both the theme of normalizing ADRD symptoms or attributing them to past trauma might be seen as manifestation of mental illness label avoidance among those who did participate in the study.

Implications for Enhancing Recruitment

Our field data drawn from multiple sources highlight several key issues affecting the recruitment of Chinese-American caregivers and their providers into studies of dementia. One issue has to do with ADRD symptom attribution. Ascribing external or normative causes to mental illness is widely recognized by clinicians as an attempt to deflect social stigma (Lefley, 1990). Although stigmatization of mental illness and of the individuals labeled with mental illness exists in most societies, the rationale behind stigmatization varies from culture to culture. In examining the causes of social stigmatization of three age-related health problems including dementia in American society, Herskovits and Mitteness (1994) found that the transgression of American values of mastery, productivity, self-control and individual responsibility results in increased social stigma to the individual. In American society where independence and individuality are prized, loss of autonomy is especially stigmatizing and to be avoided. In a less individualistic, more 'sociocentric' culture such as China's, stigmatization is imposed on the family rather than just the individual (Fabrega, 1991; Kleinman, 1986; Lee, 1982; Li & Lin, 1981; Phillips, 1993), and stems from a violation of moral virtues such as filial piety (respect and care for one's family members emphasized in Confucianism). In other words, mental illness is regarded as a punishment for violating Confucian norms governing interpersonal relations (Li & Lin, 1981). Families of mentally ill individuals may be viewed as morally corrupt. Thus normalizing ADRD symptoms might be seen as one expression of the caregiver's care—physical, social, and moral—for both the elder and the family. Our encounters with Chinese American caregivers suggested to us that as long as the caregiver felt capable of providing care, he/she saw nothing to be gained by participating in a dementia study, and only the potential for loss in the form of stigma.

The implications of the social stigma of mental illness seemed so profound that Chinese American health care providers in this study viewed protecting ADRD patients and their families from stigma as a central component of the care they provided. Providers viewed diagnosis as warranted only when violent behavior was present and/ or when they believed the family was incapable of providing adequate care (which rarely happened). In this study, only when families reached a crisis point, either in their ability to deal with their elder's increasing dependency or due to contentious family conflicts over caregiving arrangements, did they seek a formal diagnosis. These were also the families who chose to participate in the study. For these families, the strain of caregiving outweighed the potential strain of stigmatization. Although stigma was an issue for caregivers from other cultural groups participating in the study (African American, Irish American, and Latino), it seemed to operate more as an impediment to social support than to recruitment. African American and Latino caregivers, in particular, discussed concealing the elder's dementia from church communities, friends, and neighbors (Levkoff et al., in press; Reynoso, 1998). However, stigma did not emerge as such a prominent theme in recruitment interviews with caregivers from the other groups as it did with Chinese American caregivers and providers.

Strategies for Enhancing Recruitment

Effectively communicating the benefits of study participation to gatekeepers, such as health care providers, seemed to us to be crucial to recruitment success with Chinese American participants. Despite our efforts to do so, we discovered relatively late in the project that providers did not necessarily view potential benefits in the same ways in which we did. While we saw better knowledge of the disease and information about the ways in which families might be affected by it as benefits of participation, providers viewed benefits as limited to crisis management for families. An important recruitment lesson learned was that gatekeepers may share cultural biases about research with their constituents, and that extensive dialogue with them about their views of research may be necessary to establish a truly collaborative working relationship. Levkoff and colleagues (2000) note that researchers may also want to offer gatekeepers themselves tangible benefits in exchange for their collaborative support.

Inviting gatekeepers and providers to participate in the research can also strengthen recruitment efforts. Of particular value may be the involvement of gatekeepers in discussions with potential participants about confidentiality. The shared cultural understanding between Chinese American gatekeepers and potential participants of the impact of stigmatization may make gatekeeper assurances of confidentiality to participants more credible. Assurances about confidentiality and other procedural issues from Chinese American participants themselves may also help in the recruitment of other participants. For example, the knowledge that there are other Chinese American caregivers in the neighborhood struggling with the demands of caregiving and worries about stigmatization may offer some solace to caregivers. Contact with other Chinese American caregivers may help in the building of Chinese social networks in which dementia is not stigmatized. Furthermore, another caregiver attesting to the benefits of study participation may be even more persuasive than assurances coming from a gatekeeper. One last lesson we learned from this project is that the research institution needs to have credibility with community members. Our failure to recruit many caregivers through providers may have not only reflected cultural differences between us and providers on what would benefit caregiving families, but also may have reflected doubts about the sincerity of Harvard's interest in the community (see Levkoff et al., this issue). Ongoing contributions from research communities to minority communities, extending beyond the duration of a given study, may help dispel distrust.

In sum, the label of dementia proved to be a powerful obstacle to the recruitment of Chinese American research participants. It limited the effectiveness of memory screenings as a recruitment tool. It truncated recruitment conversations to such an extent that we were usually unable to fully discuss the benefits of participation with potential participants. And it limited the degree of collaboration offered by gatekeepers. Aside from following recruitment recommendations above, dementia researchers may also need to provide (or work with Alzheimer's organizations in providing) considerably more public health education about dementia to Chinese American communities in order to reduce its social stigma and increase the likelihood of recruitment success.

REFERENCES

Bhugra, D. (1989). Attitudes toward mental illness. *Acta Psychiatrica Scandinavica, 80,* 1-12.

Caban, C. (1995). Hispanic research implications of the National Institutes of Health guidelines on inclusion of women and minorities in clinical research. *Monographs of the National Cancer Institute, 18,* 165-169.

Elliott, K. S., Di Minno, M., Lam, D., & Tu, A. M. (1996). Working with Chinese families in the context of dementia. In G. Yeo & D. Gallagher-Thompson (Eds.), *Ethnicity and the dementias* (pp. 89-108). Washington, DC: Taylor & Francis.

Fabrega, H. J. (1991). Psychiatric stigma in non-Western societies. *Comprehensive Psychiatry, 32,* 534-551.

Grinnell, R. M. (1994). *Social work research and evaluation.* Itasca, IL: Peacock.

Herskovits, E. J., & Mitteness, L. S. (1994). Transgressions and sickness in old age. *Journal of Aging Studies, 8,* 327-340

Hicks, M., & Lam, M. (in press). Decision-making within the social course of dementia: Accounts by Chinese American caregivers. *Culture, Medicine, and Psychiatry.*

Hinton, W. L., & Levkoff, S. (in press). Narratives of lost identities, confusion, and loneliness in old age. *Culture, Medicine, and Psychiatry.*

Ikels, C. (1998). The experience of dementia in China. *Culture, Medicine and Psychiatry, 22,* 257-283.

Kleinman, A. (1980). *Patients and healers in the context of culture.* Berkeley: University of California.

Kleinman, A. (1986). *Social origins of distress and disease: Depression, neurasthenia, and pain in modern China.* New Haven, CT: Yale University.

Lee, E. (1982). A social systems approach to assessment and treatment in Chinese American families. In M. McGoldrick, J. K. Parce, & J. Giordano (Eds.), *Ethnicity and family therapy* (pp. 527-551). New York: Guilford.

Lefley, H. (1990). Culture and chronic mental illness. *Hospital and Community Psychiatry, 41,* 277-285.

Li, C. M. (1986). *Mind, body, and illness in Chinese medical tradition.* Unpublished doctoral dissertation, Harvard University, Cambridgr, MA.

Li, T. Y., & Lin, M. C. (1981). Love, denial and rejection: Responses of Chinese families to mental illness. In A. Kleinman & T. Lin (Eds.), *Normal and abnormal behavior in Chinese culture* (pp. 250-257). Norwell, MA: Reidel.

Levkoff, S., Levy, B., & Weitzman, P. F. (2000). The matching model of recruitment. *Journal of Mental Health and Aging, 6,* 29-38.

Levkoff, S., Levy, B., & Weitzman, P. F. (in press). The role of ethnicity and religion in the help-seeking of family caregivers. *Journal of Cross-Cultural Gerontology.*

Luborsky, M. R. (1994). The identification of themes and patterns. In J. Gubrium & A. Sankar (Eds.), *Qualitative methods in aging research* (pp. 189-210). Thousand Oaks, CA: Sage.

Mansouri, L., & Dowell, D. (1989). Perceptions of stigma among the long-term mentally ill. *Psychosocial Rehabilitation Journal, 13,* 79-91.

Phillips, M. R. (1993). Strategies used by Chinese families in coping with schizophrenia. In D. Davis & S. Harrell (Eds.), *Chinese families in the post Mao era* (pp. 277-306). Berkeley: University of California.

Rabin, R., Rosser, B., & Butler, C. (1993). Impact of diagnosis on utilities assigned to states of illness. *Journal of the Royal Society of Medicine, 86,* 439-448.

Reynoso, H. (1998, November). *Radio call-in support group for Latino caregivers.* Paper presented at the annual meeting of the Gerontological Society of America, Philadelphia, PA.

Rush, J. (1996) *Clinical anthropology: An application of anthropological concepts within clinical setting.* Westport, CT: Praeger

Tseng, W. S. (1995). The nature of somatic complaints among psychiatric patients: The Chinese case. *Comprehensive Psychiatry, 16,* 237-178.

Wang, Q. (1989). *Aging and Chinese medicine.* Sheng-Yang, China: Liang-Ling Scientific Press.

Weitzman, P. F., Chee, Y. K., & Levkoff, S. E. (1999). A social cognitive examination of responses to family conflicts by African-American and Chinese-American caregivers. *American Journal of Alzheimer's Disease.*

Young, R. F., Edevie, S., Young, J. H., & Peters, J. (1996). Issues of recruitment and retention in Alzheimer's research among African and White Americans. *Journal of Aging and Ethnicity, 1,* 19-26.

Acknowledgment. This research was conducted under the auspices of the Exploratory Center for Minority Aging and Health Promotion supported by the National Institute on Aging (Grant # P20 AG12057) and the Office for Research on Minority Health of the National Institutes of Health.

Offprints. Requests for offprints should be directed to Zibin Guo, PhD, Department of Sociology, Anthropology, and Geography, 308 Brock Hall, University of Tennessee, Chattanooga, TN 37403.

Made in the USA
Monee, IL
13 September 2026

62977347R10066